VOLUME I

COLOR ATLAS OF CERAMO-METAL TECHNOLOGY

By

Masahiro Kuwata

Visiting Professor,

Boston University

Henry M. Goldman

School of Graduate Dentistry

Boston, Massachusetts

Ishiyaku EuroAmerica, Inc.

St. Louis • Tokyo

1986

Editor in Chief: Monika E. Strong, D.D.S.
Associate Professor
Washington University
School of Dental Medicine
St. Louis, Missouri

Copy Editor: Brian Cochran M.F.A.

Make-Up Editor: Takashi Tachibana

Ishiyaku EuroAmerica, Inc.
11559 Rock Island Court, St. Louis, Missouri 63043

Library of Congress Catalogue Card Number 85-081277

Masahiro Kuwata
Color Atlas of Ceramo-Metal Technology

ISBN 0-912791-12-8

Ishiyaku EuroAmerica, Inc.   Composition by The Opticomm Group, St. Louis, Missouri
St. Louis • Tokyo   Printed in Japan

FOREWORD

Since the subject of this text is primarily the complete restoration of lost tooth structure, the reader (dental practitioner and/or dental technician) will find information here regarding many aspects of restorative dentistry. This includes most of the fundamental techniques that govern our procedures for restorative treatment of the human dentition.

The author believes that a dental practitioner or technician who is trained well and familiar with the basic techniques of restoring lost tooth structure, will not encounter any major problems in this text, even when confronted with unfamiliar or very specific types of restorative procedures. The techniques and cases shown reflect the experiences and invaluable information gathered during my visits to the United States. Since my first visit more than ten years ago, I have returned many times to observe the development of new techniques and materials. Although we must understand new developments and strive for the constant broadening of our professional horizons, I want to emphasize here that our basic restorative techniques still remain valid. They must be understood by, and taught to, both present and future professionals.

Since I entered the field of dental technology more than thirty years ago, I have had the good fortune to meet many teachers and colleagues, some of them outstanding in their professions, and to have developed many strong friendships. On this occasion, I want to extend my heartfelt gratitude to some of these men and women.

First, I want to thank Dr. C. H. Schuyler, sometimes called the father of occlusion. When I first visited the United States, the principles of occlusion were just gaining increased attention. I then met Dr. Schuyler in 1964; the professional guidance he offered me has had an enormous influence on my work.

In addition I want to thank Dr. S. Katz, one of the most important scientists in the field of ceramic materials. I met Dr. Katz and Mrs. Katz — who is also a dental technician — in 1963, when ceramic techniques were making great progress.

I would like to extend my gratitude to Dr. S. Wagman, whom I also met in 1963. He had made major contributions to the concept of restoring tooth structure in relation to crown contour, transition form, and their influence on gingival tissues. Further I want to thank Dr. R.S. Stein, whom I met in 1966. Dr. Stein taught me the biology which is so important in pontic design when restoring lost tooth structure with fixed partial dentures. He also helped me to obtain a position as Guest Lecturer/Visiting Professor at Boston University.

Furthermore, I want to thank Dr. P.E. Dawson, who gave me many important suggestions for the clinical application of group function occlusion. Finally I want to extend my gratitude to Dr. P.K. Thomas, who gave me the opportunity to study occluson just when I became interested in that great field. To this day, I can recall my excitement upon attending his occlusion course in 1965.

I also would like to extend my thanks to my dear friends Dr. R.M. Contino, Dr. R.E. Goldstein, Dr. A. Koper, Dr. S. Yuodelis, Dr. J.D. Preston, Dr. R. Sozio, Dr. L.L. Miller, Dr. S. Bergen, Dr. H.N. Yamada, and Dr. J.W. Cherberg.

Last, but not least, my special thanks to Dr. Monika E. Strong for all her efforts in editing this text and to Mr. Sanro Miwa, an original Japanese editor, who has helped me a great deal and to my photographer, Mr. Kazutomo Haraguchi.

To my parents Toshiro and Kimi Kuwata and my wife Hiroko, our children Keiko and Keiichiro, and to the staff of the Kuwata Institute, without whose support, this book could not have been written.

Masahiro Kuwata

TABLE OF CONTENTS

1

THE WORKING POSITION OF THE DENTAL TECHNICIAN: DIGITAL MANIPULATION

Manual skills, especially digital manipulation, are of great importance in the successful completion of a dental technician's daily tasks, influencing both the quality and speed of performance. The laboratory technician must possess good psychomotor skills in order to carry out the wide range of laboratory procedures, required by different projects. But unless we provide the technician with a systematic training program, focusing on both the development of psychomotor skills and of proper techniques, we cannot expect him or her to successfully complete complex tasks.

Even individuals naturally endowed with psychomotor skills will fail without adequate theoretical knowledge. For that reason, a dental technician's knowledge cannot be considered fully developed unless he or she is scientifically trained, with a gradual exposure to ergonometrics, the dynamics of instrumentation, and physiologic considerations such as the muscle tonus of the specific muscles utilized routinely in laboratory work. All of these basic concepts will be discussed here in detail.

This chapter will also analyse the various types of digital manipulation used in dental techniques and will try to derive from these the common denominators involved in the fabrication of ceramometal crowns and fixed partial dentures. Although the discussion is based on the author's experience, he hopes that it will be of value to other dentists and technicians who want to improve their individual methods by considering some of his suggestions.

1.1 THE HEIGHT OF THE WORKING TABLE AND THE THREE PRINCIPAL WORKING POSITIONS

1.1.1 THE HEIGHT OF THE WORKING TABLE

The positioning of the technician is important and should be considered from an ergonometric viewpoint. It must allow for the following:
1. Comfort and ease of work flow
2. The precise execution of the laboratory project
3. Absolute comfort for the technician, avoiding fatigue even when sitting in the same position for an extended period of time

In order to meet those requirements, the technician has to consider such factors as the type and size of the working table; the equipment it will carry; and the amount, range, and type of lighting used. In short, the technician must create a satisfactory working environment.

Clearly, the height of the work bench must be a principal consideration for the technician. When selecting a working table, consideration must first be given to the specific function for which it is intended. An office table, for example, which functions primarily as a writing space, should differ in height from a table used for pouring plaster models or carving. If the working table is too low, the technician is likely to place his elbows or other portions of the forearm in a manner that will interfere with proper work flow. In the author's opinion, the optimal working table must permit the technician to be seated deeply and comfortably in his chair while not further than approximately 25 cm. away from any one work project. The technician's wrists should be lightly supported by the table's edge. The height of the working table is dictated by the size of the person using it. Since the average height of the Japanese male is 5'6", we recommend that the table be 32-33.5 inches high. Any adjustment of the table's height must be followed by an adjustment of the accompanying chair, whose foot rest should also be adjustable to permit comfortable positioning of the legs.

1.1.2 THREE PRINCIPAL WORKING POSITIONS

Note: Most technicans are right-handed. That fact, therefore, will receive priority attention.

Basic Position No. 1

The head is bent slightly forward and the handrest established on the table with the outer edge of the right hand (and sometimes with the finger tips of the left hand). In this position the technician is working bimanually.

Basic Position No. 2

When a procedure is performed without a handrest, the chin is retracted slightly, and — by placing the forearms lightly on the table, with the wrists somewhat away from the edge — the technician can work comfortably.

Basic Position No. 3

A rest is established by placing the left wrist lightly on the table edge. Thus minute work can be performed while instruments are held with the right hand and working models with the left. Although some procedures demand a standing working position, most dental techniques can be performed in any of the three above-described positions, with occasional minor changes, depending on the size and type of the the projects being worked on. Remember that when maintaining any of the above working positions, no unnecessary stress is exerted upon the spinal column and shoulders unless the neck is unduly bent. By reducing strain, which is counterproductive, greater strength and efficiency result. It is important to sit straight and deep in the chair. The technician who sits at a 90 degree position is less likely to violate the concepts of human engineering. Any other position reduces the technician's concentration upon his task. Good work positioning habits are imperative in avoiding stress and fatigue.

**THREE REQUIREMENTS FOR
THE WORKING POSITION**

1. The position must allow the technician to work comfortably.
2. The position must permit the performance of precision work.
3. The position must create minimum fatigue and permit working conditions for extended periods of time.

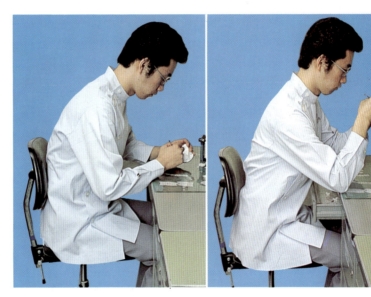

The height of the working table is crucial in avoiding fatigue. If too low, as in the illustration on the left, the technician tends to bend forward. If too high, on the other hand, the elbows tend to rest on the table, as in the illustration on the right.

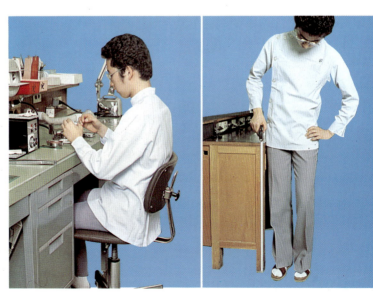

When the technician is seated in his chair and his project is within a range of vision of about 25 cm, both wrists rest lightly on the edge of the table and provide complete freedom for his hands. The illustration on the right shows a 32″ high working table. The technician is 5′6″ tall.

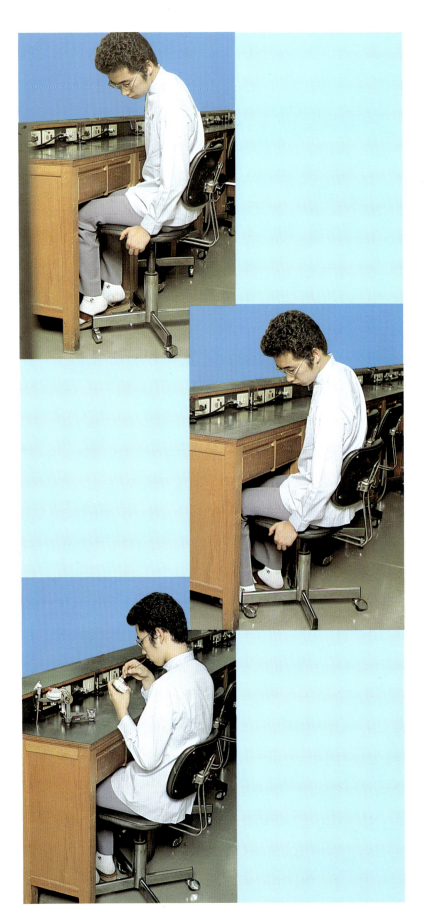

A foot rest is used to adjust the sitting height of the technician.

Above: The heels are up in the air.

Center: The heels are on the floor.

Below: A 90-degree position.

The height of the working table is adjusted to allow for maximum effectiveness of the technician. Again, let us review the three principal working positions mentioned above.

THREE PRINCIPAL WORKING POSITIONS

Basic Position No. 1:   The head is bent slightly forward and the handrest established on the table with the outer edge of the right hand (and sometimes with the finger tips of the left hand). In this position the technician is working bi-manually.

Basic Position No. 2:   When a procedure is performed without a handrest, the chin is retracted slightly, and — by placing the forearms lightly on the table, with the wrists somewhat away from the edge — the technician can work comfortably.

Basic Position No. 3:   A rest is established by placing the left wrist lightly on the table edge. Thus minute work can be performed while instruments are held with the right hand and working models with the left.

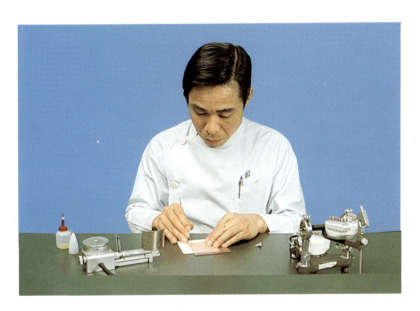

Basic position No. 1, in which sheet wax is being cut on the table.

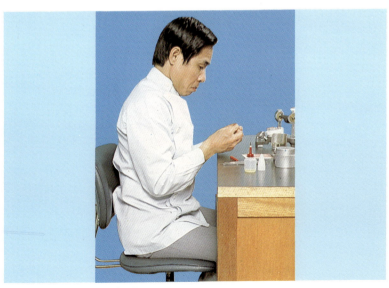

Basic position No. 2, in which all ten fingers are coordinated to carry out a task.

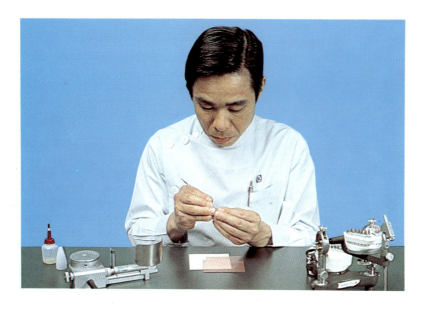

Basic position No. 3, in which detailed carving procedures are performed with a carving instrument.

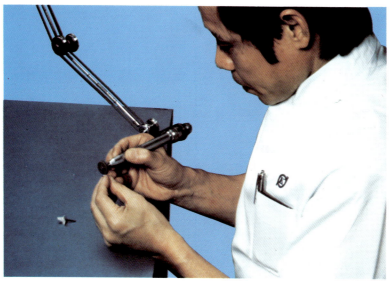

A task which necessitates the application of strong force is performed in position No. 3, while detailed procedures, performed with a minimum expenditure of force, are best accomplished in position No. 2.

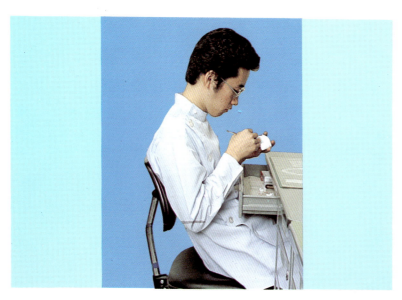

This illustration shows an undesirable working position which results in fatigue.

1.2 PRINCIPAL WORKING POSITIONS AND DIGITAL MANIPULATION

In any type of manual activity, coordination of the hands and fingers takes place on more or less an unconscious level. But if we watch a dental technician at work, we will notice certain recurrent patterns controlling his finger movements: in cutting a sheet of wax, for example, the technician's repetitive activity requires a trained coordination of the fingers. In this section, we will discuss digital manipulation in conjunction with basic working positions.

The terminology associated with digital manipulation:

Fixation: (Handrest, fingerest)	The positioning of the wrists and fingers to stabilize the project on the work table
Hold:	The finger positioning that holds the project in place
Retention: (Stabilization)	The finger positioning that stabilizes the hands and, at the same time, frees the working fingers
Handling:	The finger positioning for proper instrument handling
Operation:	The basic finger movement for any manipulation (operating or working fingers)

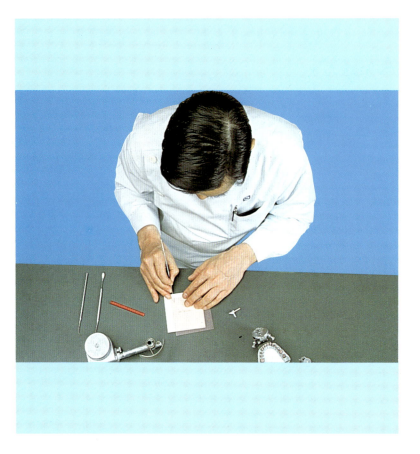

Fingers in basic working position No. 1.

To use basic working position No. 1 correctly the sheet wax must be placed on the table within the operator's full range of vision. If the sheet wax is placed too far away from the technician, he is apt to bend forward, resulting in fatigue. The portion of the sheet wax to be cut should be nearly under the corner of the right eye. During this procedure, the five fingers of the left hand hold the sheet wax in place. The thumb, index, and middle finger of the right hand then hold the instrument at 90 degree angle for lateral movement, and at about 45 degrees for forward and backward movement.

The ring and little fingers steady the right hand on the table and provide stability for the carving instrument in motion.

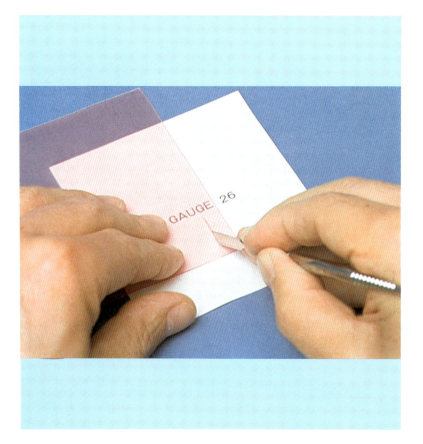

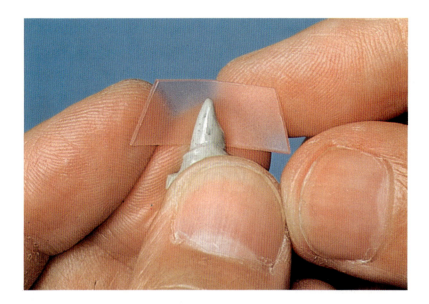

Working in basic position No. 2.

In basic position No. 2, fixation is not obtained on the table. This shall be illustrated with the manipulation of a piece of sheet wax.

The procedure is performed with the fingers only, involving no instrument. Both elbows are held lightly against the body, and the wrists kept slightly away from the table's edge while the project is brought within the technician's sight. By holding the tips of the middle, ring, and little fingers together, the sheet wax is pressed from the proximal tooth surface to the lingual and buccal sides of the die, so an effort can be made to closely adapt the wax to the die. As this procedure progresses, the tip of the right thumb and the bottom of the left index finger are used to close the open ends of the sheet wax.

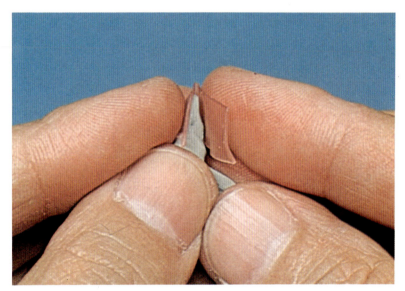

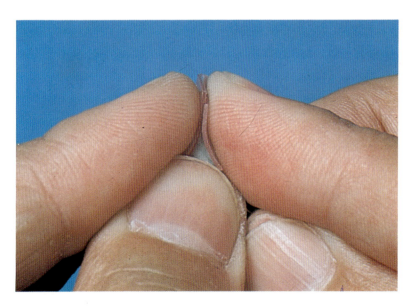

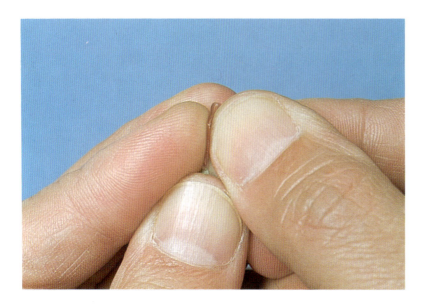

1. The technician can retain the die in the tips of the right thumb and the left index finger, thus stabilizing and immobilizing it.
2. Without arm movement, the technician's fingers remain stabilized while retaining full freedom of movement.
3. Using the right thumb and the left index finger, the technician is bringing the plastic sheet wax into close contact with the tooth for an exact impression.

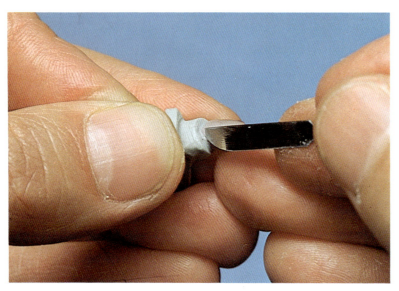

Adjustment of a die-margin in basic working position No. 3.

In this working position, one can perform a variety of tasks, such as waxing up patterns, carving, final adjustment of castings, the construction of a porcelain crown, etc. To hold the die, one should rest the hands at the front edge of the table, with the thumb, index, middle, and ring fingers holding the die. The middle finger should be extended higher than the other fingers in order to keep the sheet wax in place This serves to steady the die when its margin is cut off. Although the tips of the right ring and left middle fingers hold the model, both also stabilize it. The mutual coordination of thumb, middle, and ring fingers is identical with position No. 1.

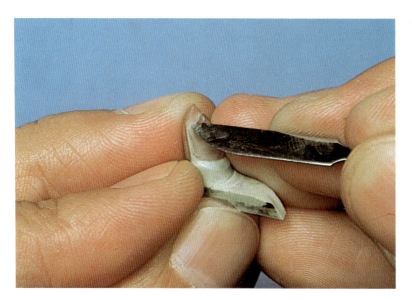

1.3 TEN PRINCIPLES OF DIGITAL MANIPULATION

For all dental procedures, the correct use of the fingers and hand instruments (which function finger-like) is essential. In conjunction with the basic working positions, a set of standardized principles has been established for digital and instrumental manipulation. The term **instrument** here refers to tools used to construct or modify materials, resulting in a prescribed form of dental restoration. An instrument may be a carving knife, brush, blade, spatula, or handpiece, but in our terminology it does not include equipment like burnout furnaces, porcelain furnaces, vacuum investors, or casting machines.

The following ten principles, then, govern digital manipulation.

No. 1 A laboratory project is placed within clear view of the operator, where he/she can accomplish the task easily without undue physical strain.

No. 2 The fingertips have to be brought into proximity with each other, especially when the project requires detailed and precise manipulation.

No. 3 When the task requires the use of both hands, they must function together in a standardized manner. Each hand is assigned a working role.

No. 4 When working unimanually, all five fingers must be assigned specific roles. When working bimanually, all ten fingers must be coordinated to perform their respective tasks.

No. 5 A functional role is assigned to each finger.

No. 6 Stability must be considered when both hands are used.

No. 7 Any operation using one hand only should be limited to the type of work which does not necessitate stability.

No. 8 For minute and detailed projects less force is transmitted to the fingertips.

No. 9 The little finger is separated from the other fingers, thus serving as a support.

No. 10 When a task requires a strong hold — cutting procedures, for instance — a supporting finger should be placed close to the working fingers.

Before any technical dental project is initiated, we must define our goals and objectives. For example:

For crown and bridge restorations the following goals have been established:

1. Preservation of the health of the gingival tissues and the entire periodontium
2. Restoration of occlusal function

In order to achieve the final goal, we must establish the required contour, the proper marginal fit, good surface finish, and the biologic transition form between crown and root surfaces. Only after these have been accomplished is it possible to restore the original phonetic and esthetic functions of the dentition in harmony with a healthy periodontal apparatus, facial features, and the natural coloration of the patient. During each step in prosthetic procedure, specific goals and objectives are accomplished, and skilled digital manipulation is imperative for their completon.

This chapter focuses on correct digital manipulation with respect to waxing techniques and the adjustment and finishing of metal alloys in the fabrication of ceramometal crowns.

TEN PRINCIPLES OF DIGITAL MANIPULATION

No. 1 A laboratory project is placed within clear view of the operator, where he/she can accomplish the task easily without undue physical strain.

No. 2 The fingertips have to be brought into proximity with each other, especially when the project requires detailed and precise manipulation.

No. 3 When the task requires the use of both hands, they must function together in a standardized manner. Each hand is assigned a working role.

No. 4 When working unimanually, all five fingers must be assigned specific roles. When working bimanually, all ten fingers must be coordinated to perform their respective tasks.

No. 5 A functional role is assigned to each finger.

No. 6 Stability must be considered when both hands are used.

No. 7 Any operation using one hand only should be limited to the type of work which does not necessitate stability.

No. 8 For minute and detailed projects less force is transmitted to the fingertips.

No. 9 The little finger is separated from the other fingers, thus serving as a support.

No. 10 When a task requires a strong hold — cutting procedures, for instance — a supporting finger should be placed close to the working fingers.

The wax-up of a crown

In order to avoid wasting precious work time, care must be taken not to apply excessive wax to the die.

1) Carving off wax for adjustments will waste time and create delays. Furthermore, the added pressure exerted on the wax periphery prevents an exact fit of the margin, and tends to rotate the pattern on the die. This will happen to a greater degree the further from the center of rotation pressure is exerted (A).

2) If excessive amounts of wax are added on the occlusal surface, the pattern may be distorted toward the margin (B).

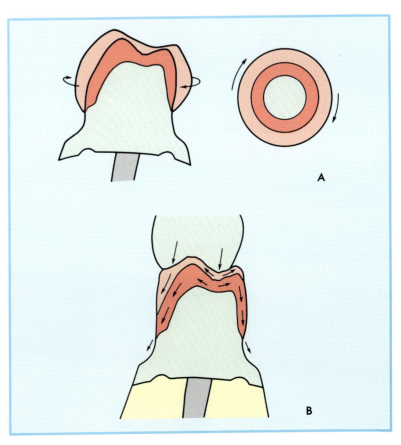

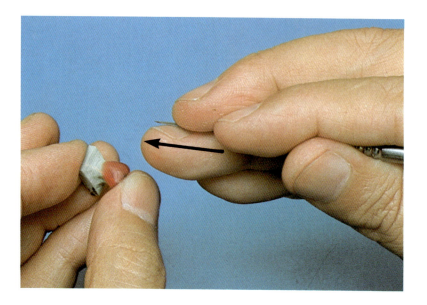

In all waxing techniques, it is most important to melt the wax at an optimal temperature since temperature control influences manipulation of the wax during construction and carving of the pattern. In this illustration, a technician confirms the working temperature by putting the tip of the carving instrument between the thumb and index finger.

This method of temperature confirmation also facilitates removal of excess wax.

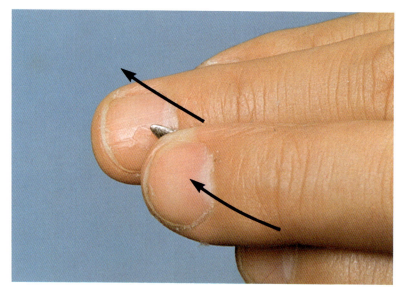

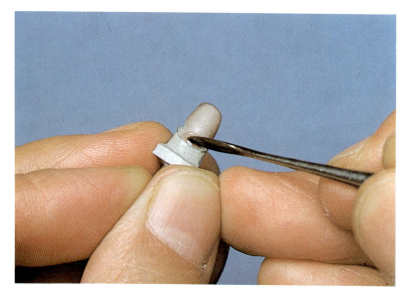

Inlay wax is being added to a die. Using basic working position No. 3, all ten fingers are fully engaged in this task.

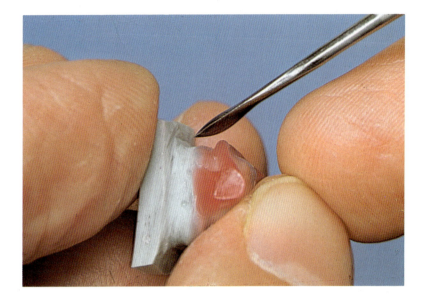

The wax-up procedure performed with both hands. The principles of finger coordination are well observed.

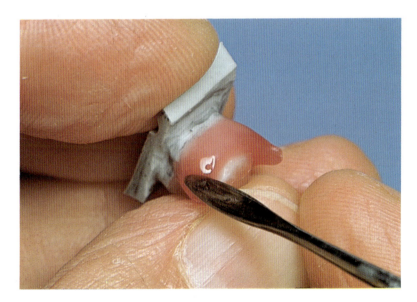

The wax is being built up and shaped at the same time. The three working fingers (thumb, index, and middle) lightly hold the carving instrument. For detailed procedures, the tip of the most sensitive finger should be employed.

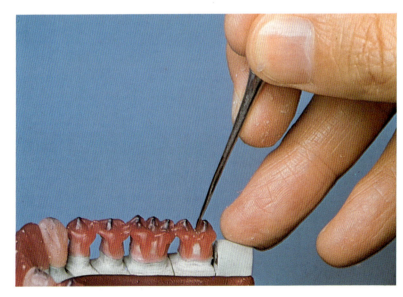

Wax is built up using only one hand. Support is maintained with the tip of the ring finger. When working with a very small amount of wax, an effort is made to apply the least amount of force possible, with the carving instrment held gently between the three working fingers. The other fingers are separated to give them freedom to move.

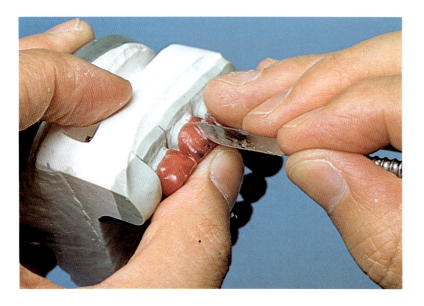

Carving wax

More force is applied to the wax pattern when carving wax. For this reason, support should be obtained with two fingers (the middle and little) for a better grasp.

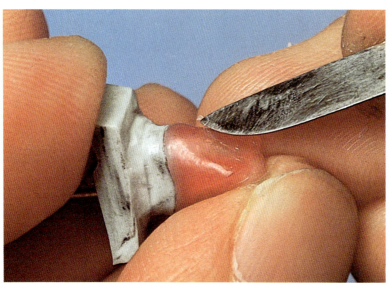

Another illustration of waxing and carving: here the lingual surface is finished with all fingers fully coordinated. During this operation, the left thumb holds the wax pattern from the occlusal-lingual surface with a force light enough to avoid distortion of the wax.

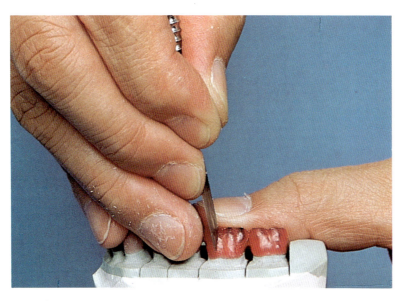

A similar procedure, showing the carving of the buccal side of the mandibular molars.

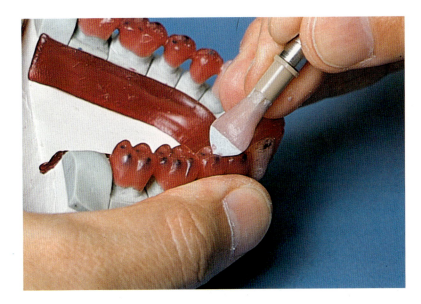

When carving the occlusal surface, the side of the wax pattern is held with the left thumb.

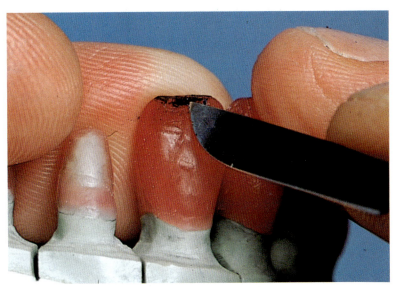

When carving the labial side of the (maxillary) canine, the lingual side of the wax pattern is held with the left middle finger.

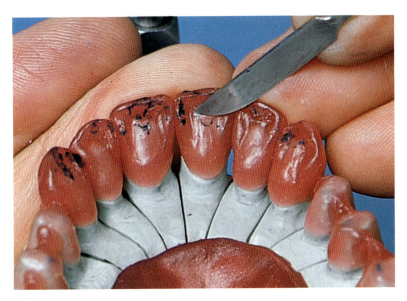

When carving the lingual side of the anterior teeth, the wax pattern is smilarly held.

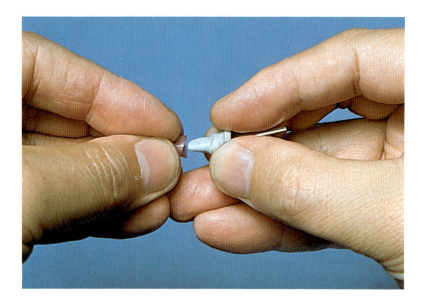

During waxing, the coping must eventually be recovered from the die. During this process, distortion of the wax pattern must be avoided at all costs. The left fingers should hold the coping while the right fingers remove the die. If the force of the fingers is not uniform, the coping will tend to be distorted or crushed, especially if two fingers are used for the removal. For this reason, the operator holds the sides of the coping with the fingers of the left hand and distributes their force evenly, while the right thumb, index, and middle fingers slide the die away from the pattern for easy removal. The right and left ring fingers can then act as a support for the operation.

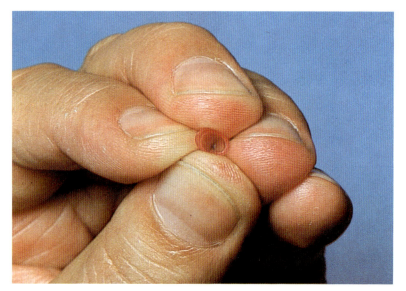

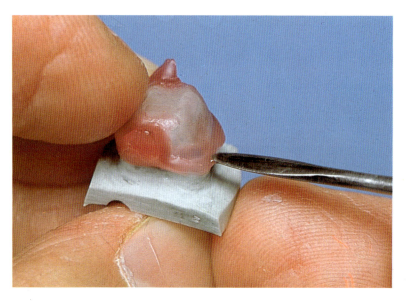

When a heated carving instrument is used for the wax-up of the pattern, subsequent carving can be reduced to a minimum. During this procedure, the three working fingers lightly hold the carving knife while the right and left ring fingers play a supporting role. Here the force of the working fingers is reduced so that the little finger can balance the supporting fingers.

Adjustment of the metal substructures.

When adjustments on a hard metal alloy are performed at high speed, basic working position No. 3 is assumed if greater force must be applied. Detailed procedures performed with less force require basic working position No. 2. The guidelines for the adjustment of a casting are identical to the ones followed with the waxing techniques:

1. If the size of the project permits, all fingers are used to hold it firmly. The thumb is positioned to counteract pressure, i.e., in the opposite direction of the pressure (basic working positions 3, 4).

2. When performing detailed tasks requiring minute control, the left thumb of the holding hand is positioned near a rotating point so that it can exert more force and be most resistant to force acting from the outside (basic working positions 2,4).

3. The project is placed in clear view, and any instruments are arranged so as not to obstruct the view (basic working positions 1,3). (page 21 and 22)

4. The adjustment of a metal alloy project requires a greater manual force than usual. Therefore, complete coordination of both hands and fingers is necessary. At the same time, the right little finger is positioned to give support to the fingers of the left hand (basic working positions 4,6,10).

5. The handpiece is held firmly with the three working fingers. When a project is detailed, the handpiece is held closer to its tip (basic working positions 2,5).

6. Of the three working fingers, the index finger directs the handpiece, the middle and ring fingers are used to stabilize it, and the thumb controls direction (basic working positions 4,5).

In instances when it is difficult to hold firmly onto a project in the absence of a sprue or other residual metal, the technician must work out some unconventional type of digital manipulation. When holding a small project, the following rules must be considered:

1. The working fingers should make the widest possible contact with the project. A strong grasp of the object gives it maximum stability.

2. The more fingers employed for holding a project, the more stable it will be.

3. The fingers should be manipulated so as not to block a clear view of the object. When working on a wide surface, using a somewhat large stone at reduced speed is more effective than using a small stone which requires many small movements. Reduced working speed also generates less friction heat. The following set of photographs illustrates cutting procedures and associated tasks involving the removal of the sprue. Aside from the varying size of the rotary cutting instruments, dependent on the project size, the principles governing digital manipulation are the same as those described previously in conjunction with working techniques.

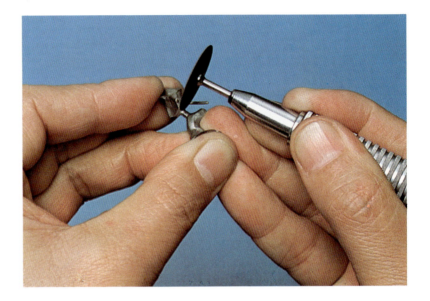

During this operation, we must prevent the cast restoration from being flung out by the rotation of the disc. The index and middle fingers of the right hand hold the casting, and the left thumb, ring, and little fingers hold the remaining sprue, with the right ring and little fingers functioning as support. To cut the sprue wire accurately, the exact position of the cutting disc must be well planned in advance.

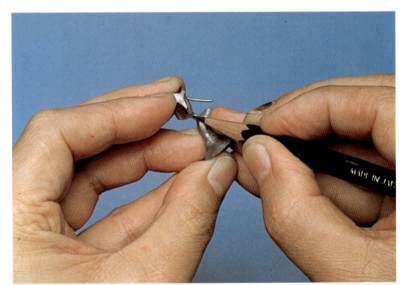

Marking the position with a pencil will help. The fingers must not block the view of the field of operation.

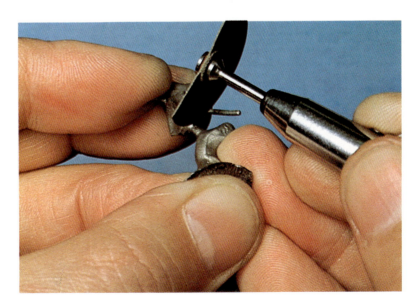

The restoration is securely held in order to avoid disc breakage. If a disc should block the operator's vision, it can be partially cut for better vision, as shown in the illustration at right. It is then possible to view the working area through the rotation of the disc.

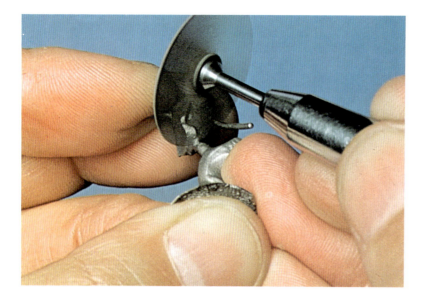

The sprue wire is cut with a partially cut disc. This method was first demonstrated by Dr. P.K. Thomas.

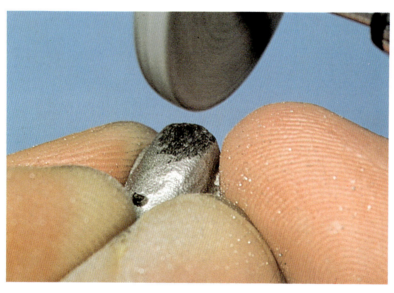

The cut surface between the sprue wire and the casting must now be finished. The goal here is to create a contact as wide as possible and to reduce its exposed surface to a minimum for any adjustment. Here the Busch Co. heatless stone is used at reduced speed to obtain a flat surface.

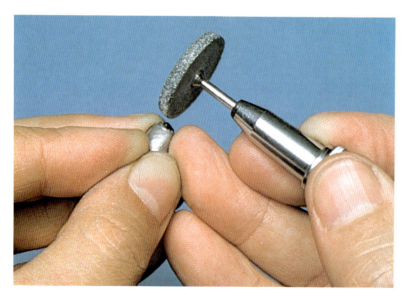

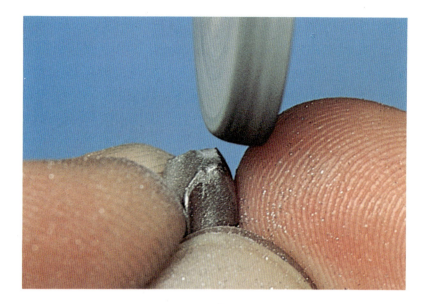

The tip of the casting is now adjusted.

Although this holding position does not adhere to the standardized pattern, the principles governing digital manipulation, the supporting hand, finger coordination, and the handling of the handpiece remain the same. A somewhat larger stone should be used for this procedure, directing the handpiece with wide strokes toward the operator.

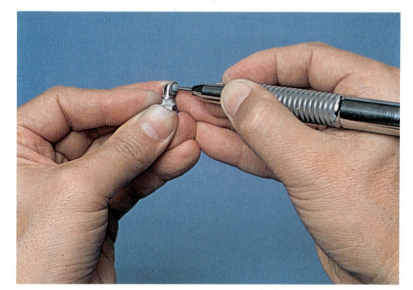

This illustration shows the adjustment of a fired porcelain surface. Note the well-balanced hand and finger coordination. Minor protuberances inside the crown are adjusted under magnification for improved precision fit.

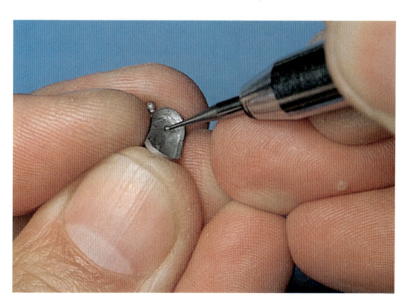

During this detailed and minute process the project should not be moved at all. In accordance with the above-mentioned principles, it is securely held in place and supported with the fingers of the left hand.

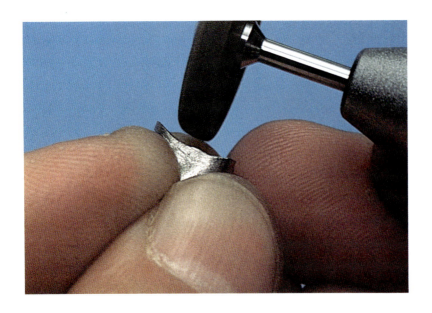

A minute adjustment on the crown margin using a porcelain finish wheel (Shofu Dental Co. P2 product).

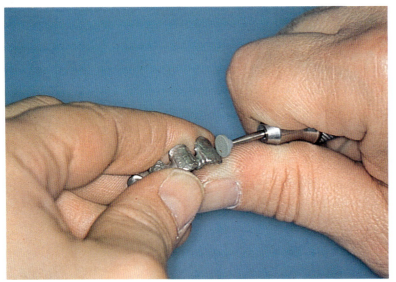

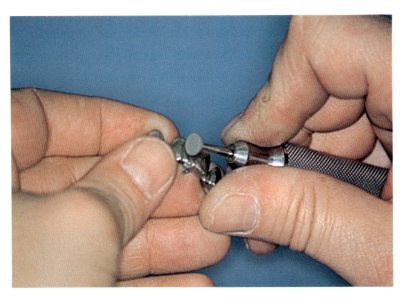

Here, we differentiate between two different grasps for handling a carving instrument: the pen grasp and the palm grasp. Although both techniques have their merit, greater force can be exercised with the palm grasp; the working project should be held as near to the finger tips as possible.

Concluding remarks

In this section some important aspects of digital manipulation in the dental laboratory have been discussed, with reference to waxing techniques and the manipulation of metal alloys. In both of these areas, well-balanced hand and finger coordination is extremely important. In alternating working techniques, the carving instrument is held with the tips of the working fingers. While the fingers of the right hand perform the main task, the left fingers play a supporting role. When finishing a crown, for example, it is necessary to hold it firmly in place. This also goes for adjusting and grinding freehand or on a model. Furthermore, throughout the waxing procedure, the wax pattern must never be detached from the die since the slightest movement during this operation could lead to a distortion of the pattern. Proper digital manipulation skills must be systematically taught to the beginning dental technician. I have often noted that even trained technicians and dentists tend to use their fingers habitually and without any theoretical and systematic background in standardized waxing techniques.

2

OBJECTIVE FOR RESTORING FORM, FUNCTION, AND ESTHETICS

The dental technician's fabrication of a cast crown can be compared to the dentist's restoration of teeth. When constructing ceramometal restorations it is important to arrive at biologically compatible restorations which achieve an optimal functional balance in terms of strength, phonetics, and esthetic appearance. The ultimate goal is to fabricate restorations which are both physiologically and esthetically satisfactory for the patient.

If a restoration should fail to meet any one of these requirements, it does not serve our purposes.

Harmony of a cast restoration with the surrounding healthy gingiva is a must. The recent introduction of a dentoform showing soft gingivae is indicative of the growing emphasis on the periodontal aspect of restorative dentistry. As a matter of fact, the contour of the gingival tissues and embrasures furnishes a valuable guide for the three-plane construction of a crown.

The present chapter focuses on the anatomically correct contour of planned cast restorations which should reproduce previously lost tooth structures.

In the construction of ceramometal fixed restorations, several requirements have to be satisfied. In addition to the need for biological harmony with the gingival tissues, the achievement of correct phonetics, and an esthetically pleasing appearance, a prosthesis has to be strong enough to withstand daily masticatory attrition and abrasion. When multiple fixed restorations are fabricated, each of the units must match the others perfectly. One defective unit causes the entire restoration to fail. We must regard the oral cavity as an entity.

**REQUIREMENTS FOR THE
CERAMOMETAL RESTORATION**

I. RESTORATION OF OCCLUSAL FUNCTION
   A. OCCLUSAL HARMONY DURING MANDIBULAR MOVEMENT
   B. RESTORATION OF THE SWALLOWING FUNCTION

II. FUNCTIONAL HARMONY WITH ADJACENT LIVING TISSUE
   A. INTEGRITY OF GINGIVAL TISSUES AND EMBRASURES
   B. PROPER MARGINAL FIT
   C. CONTOUR COMPATIBILITY WITH GINGIVAL TISSUES
   D. PROPER CONTOUR FOR SELF-CLEANSING
   E. SMOOTH SURFACE FINISH WHERE REQUIRED
   F. CROWN CONTOUR COMPATIBLE WITH THE BUCCAL, LABIAL AND LINGUAL SOFT AND HARD STRUCTURES OF THE MOUTH

III. RESISTANCE FORM
   STRENGTH OF THE CAST METAL ALLOY
   A. DESIGN STRENGTH RELATED TO ALLOY PROPERTIES
   B. BOND STRENGTH
   C. STRENGTH INFLUENCED BY MATERIAL MANIPULATION
   D. STRENGTH AS MATERIAL PROPERTY STRENGTH OF THE CERAMIC MATERIAL
   A. STRENGTH BASED ON CORRECT MANIPULATION
   B. STRENGTH OF THE CERAMIC DESIGN
   C. STRENGTH AS A MATERIAL PROPERTY COMBINED STRENGTH

IV. RESTORATION OF PHONETICS
   A. ARRANGEMENT OF TEETH
   B. CORRECT ANATOMY OF THE CROWN PORTION

V. RESTORATION OF ESTHETICS
   A. HARMONY WITH HEALTHY GINGIVAL TISSUES
   B. HARMONY BETWEEN FACIAL FEATURES AND CROWN CONTOUR
   C. RESTORATION OF NATURAL COLOURING

2.1 THE BALANCED RESTORATION OF TEETH

The balanced restoration of teeth must entail the criteria just listed. When constructing ceramometal fixed restorations, it is essential that the teeth be properly prepared in order to meet the requirements mentioned above.

The restoration(s) must be in harmony with the entire supporting apparatus. Only after this requirement is satisfactorily met can considerations of phonetic function and esthetics become meaningful. For this reason, the given requirements are closely interrelated, thus constituting an organic entity.

Since all of these requirements are organically related, the absence of even one factor will mean the failure of an otherwise adequate restoration. This is particularly true of prosthetic procedures involving multiple restorations, in which a defect of one restoration will destroy the esthetic appearance of the whole and be a detriment to oral function and to the happiness of the patient.

The requirements listed above are a summary of the goals for which a dental technician must always strive, i.e., the creation of good form and function.

Our current criterion as to whether a restoration is good or bad is partly based on the fact that a given cast restoration, cemented permanently, either maintains or impairs the health of the gingivae. This in turn relates to possible deposition of dental plaque as the main factor in periodontal disease and/or dental caries. A ceramometal restoration provides an ideal prosthetic means of meeting our criteria, since it satisfies the requirements for both form and function.

Some properties of dental porcelain
1. Porcelain is compatible with gingival tissues
2. Porcelain surfaces can be finished smoothly
3. Porcelain is abrasion resistant and does not absorb water
4. Porcelain has an excellent esthetic appearance

The criterion for judging whether a restoration is adequate or unsatisfactory consists in its harmony with existing healthy periodontium. If defective, it will contribute to the accumulation of dental plaque, which in turn will lead to periodontal disease and/or dental caries. The criteria for prevention of disease are identical with the ones for form and function (see below).

Conventional porcelains do not possess sufficient strength to be used alone, but must be fused with a metal-alloy.

Because of problems such as poorly fitting substructures, poor contour, and lack of smoothness at the cervical region combined with possible irritation of the gingivae, ceramometal restorations have not been given the recognition which they deserve. Many of those problems, however, are a function of the dental technician's work, so with sufficient training, they can be readily surmounted.

When constructing cast restorations, it is important to realize that lost or prepared portions of the tooth/teeth are replaced. If we use multiple materials such as metal-alloys combined with opaque and porcelains of various shades, it is imperative to know how they will perform under regular wear. The failure of ceramometal restorations often derives from a poor understanding of the materials used — their properties and correct manipulation. In the present chapter, the integrity of the gingival tissues and crown contour shall be discussed in this context.

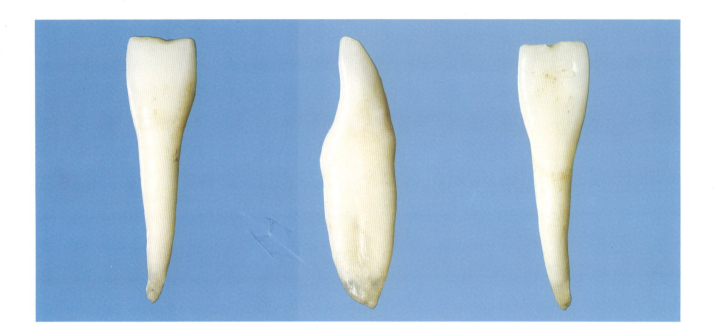

An extracted natural tooth is examined from various sides. It is evident that there are no sharp angles on the surfaces of a natural tooth. For this reason, an artificial restoration should also have a biologically acceptable transition form from crown to root surface.

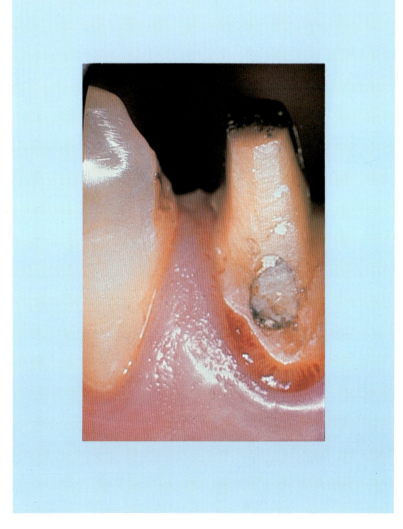

This photograph shows an invasion of some tissue at the gingival margin, an area which must be given primary consideration when planning ceramometal restorations (photograph courtesy of Dr. R.S. Stein). The causes of this type of distortion are twofold: either they begin in the wax-up process (and the investing and casting) or they are traceable to the heat treatment of the cast alloy and the subsequent firing of the porcelain. Therefore, it is necessary that metals least subject to distortion by heat be selected for ceramometal restorations.

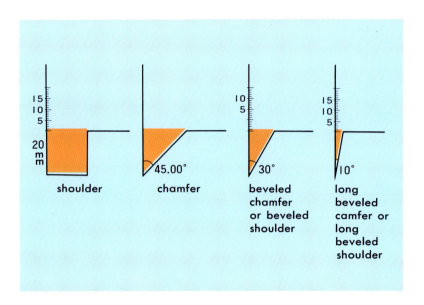

Expansion of the luting cement accounts for the failure to seat a crown and is directly related to the chamfer angle of the gingival margin. In clinical situations, the relationship between the space at the gingival margin and a gingival chamfer of the crown preparation is determined by the chamfer of the crown and the inclination of the abutment tooth.

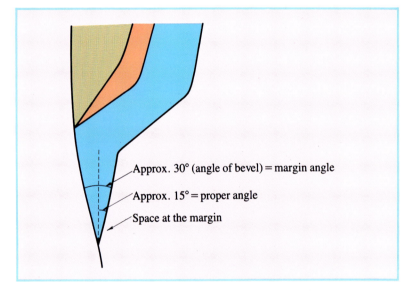

Approx. 30° (angle of bevel) = margin angle

Approx. 15° = proper angle

Space at the margin

	100 μm	90 μm	80 μm	70 μm	60 μm	50 μm	40 μm	30 μm	20 μm	10 μm
10°	17.360	15.624	13.888	12.152	10.416	8.680	6.944	5.208	3.472	1.736
20°	34.200	30.780	27.360	23.940	20.520	17.100	13.680	10.260	6.840	3.420
30°	50.000	45.000	40.000	35.000	30.000	25.000	20.000	15.000	10.000	5.000
40°	64.280	57.852	51.424	44.996	38.568	32.140	25.710	19.280	12.850	6.428
50°	76.600	68.940	61.280	53.620	45.960	38.300	30.640	22.980	15.320	7.660
60°	86.600	77.940	69.280	60.620	51.960	43.300	34.640	25.980	17.320	8.660
70°	93.970	84.573	75.175	65.779	56.382	46.980	37.580	28.190	18.790	9.397
80°	98.480	88.632	78.784	68.936	59.088	49.240	39.390	29.540	19.690	9.848
90°	100.000	90.000	80.000	70.000	60.000	50.000	40.000	30.000	20.000	10.000

The following table gives the correlation between crown chamfers and amounts of crown taper.

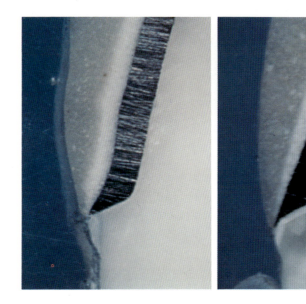

By furnishing a beveled chamfer, it is possible to keep tooth reduction at the margin to a minimum. However, when this is undesirable from an esthetic viewpoint, the marginal reduction must be carried deeper. The left view shows a crown, (representing the mean out of 100) constructed after using a die spacer: at right we see a crown fabricated without using a die spacer.

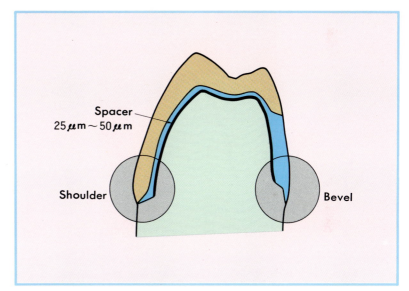

The possible necessity for coating the die with a spacer (and determination of its thickness) is determined by the following criterion: when abutment teeth are long and their taper is minimal, the coating of the die must compensate for the excessively tight fit of the crown.

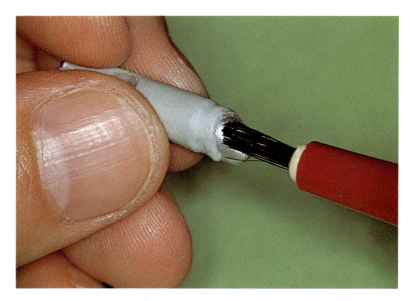

Of the many spacers available, our selection should be based on uniform coating effect, ease in determining thickness, and adhesion to the die during the waxing process.

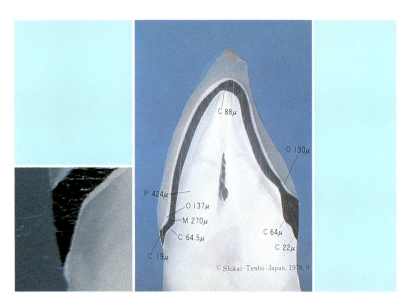

© Shikai–Tenbo (Japan, 1978. 9)

A bevel of about 25° is established with a convenient bevel of about 15°. The amount of space at the labial margin is 19μm without use of a spacer. The exposed metal part shows a smooth continuation of the root surface.

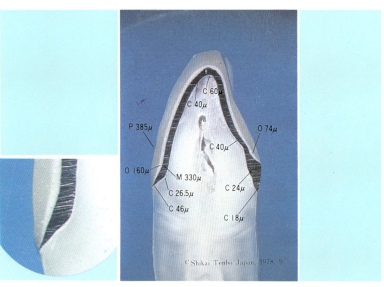

© Shikai Tenbo Japan, 1978. 9

A chamfer type without bevel, where a conformable bevel is 50°. The amount of space at the labial margin is 46μm without use of a spacer. When compared with the illustration above, this restoration does not fit as accurately at the chamfer area. Here, the margin is well covered with a combination of metal, opaque, and porcelain components. Its transition to the root surface is also favorable.

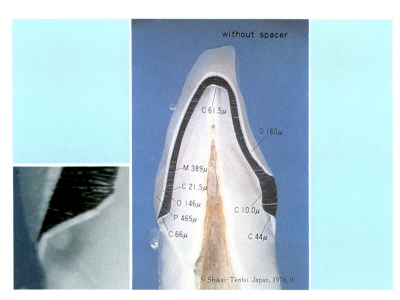

without spacer

© Shikai–Tenbo (Japan, 1978. 9)

A shoulder type without bevel, where a conformable bevel is 70°. The amount of space at the labial margin is 66μm, without use of a spacer. Since the crown fit is much reduced by an increased chamfer, the use of a spacer is recommended. In this case, however, satisfactory coverage is guaranteed through the proper combinaton of materials used.

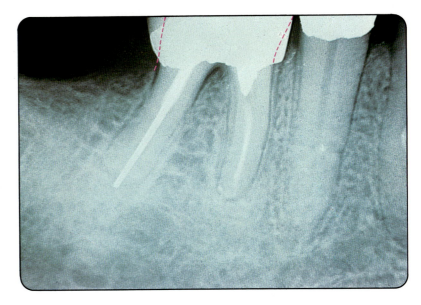

Here the desirable smooth transition from the restoration to the root is missing. This results in gross overcontour of the restoration. In this case, the crown should be contoured mesiodistally, as indicated by the dotted line. Even at the expense of the distal cusp of the third molar, the periodontal health of this tooth should be considered a priority (photograph courtesy of Dr. R.S. Stein).

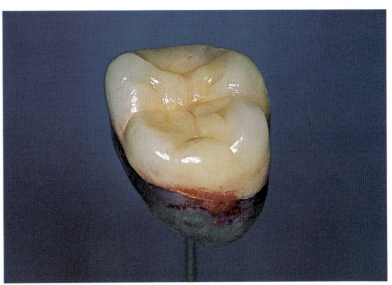

To prove the point illustrated in the photograph above, a crown was fabricated for the author's mandibular right second molar. It was purposely overcontoured, especially distally. This crown was subsequently placed into the author's mouth and left there for a period of several months. During this time it proved impossible to maintain proper oral hygiene in that area (illustration courtesy of Dr. K. Marumori).

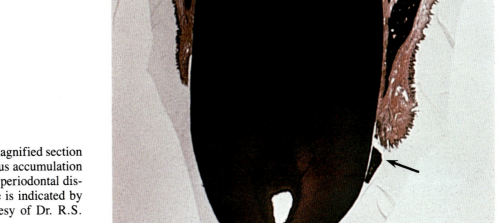

This illustration shows a magnified section of a dissected tooth. Calculous accumulation at the gingival sulcus causes periodontal disease; the calculous area here is indicated by an arrow (photograph courtesy of Dr. R.S. Stein).

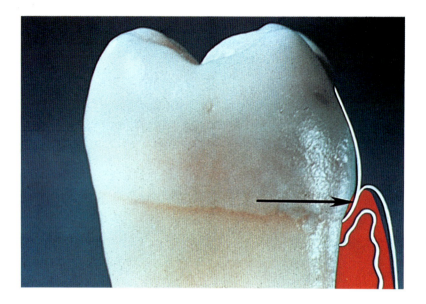

When a crown is overcontoured, it will not only interfere with proper oral health but will also impinge on the gingiva, where poor blood circulation will cause gingival inflammation, subsequently affecting the entire periodontal apparatus (photograph courtesy of Dr R.S. Stein).

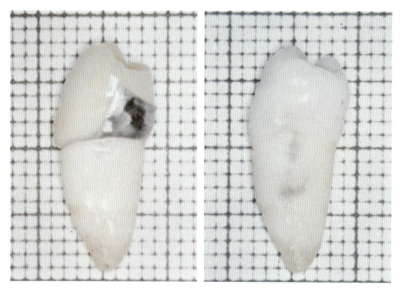

The left side shows an overcontoured crown; at right we can see the anatomical contour of an extracted tooth. It is important not to exceed the anatomical contour. When the preparation depth and chamfer angle are executed correctly, it is possible to achieve a smooth transition from crown to root surface without overcontouring. If these factors are not observed at the beginning of the preparation, any effort to cover the margin with porcelain will result in overcontour.

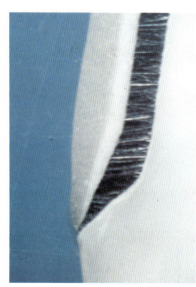
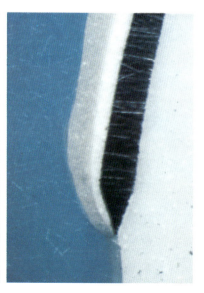

Left: This illustration shows how adequate shoulder preparation guarantees, without overcontouring, correct distribution of the three materials involved in crown construction.

Right: This illustration gives an enlarged dissected view of the overcontoured crown shown in center left. Note the incorrect angulation of the shoulder preparation and the ensuing problem. This refers to the triangular theory.

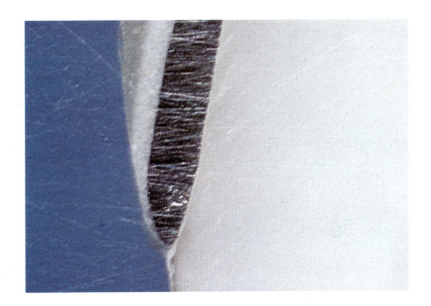

This view shows the exposure of opaque material on the lingual surface boundary between the porcelain and metal. Regardless of how the opaque material is heated and polished it is impossible for it to reach the necessary smoothness of fired and finished porcelain.

An opaque line is exposed on the labial margin because of deficient preparation depth at the camfer.

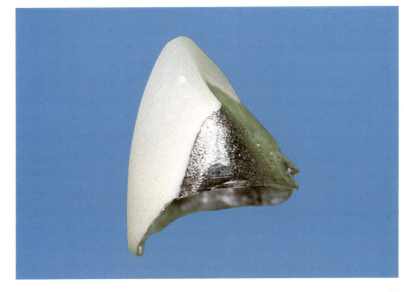

Exposed opaque material in the proximal area and labial margin. When exposed opaque comes into contact with the gingiva, plaque is deposited in the area and gingival tissues are constantly irritated, leading to peridontal disease.

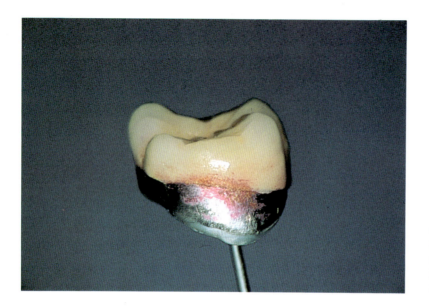

A porcelain crown with an incompletely condensed and glazed surface and a porous (thus inadequately finished) metal part. Adequate contour and finish of the surface are important in the prevention of plaque deposition.

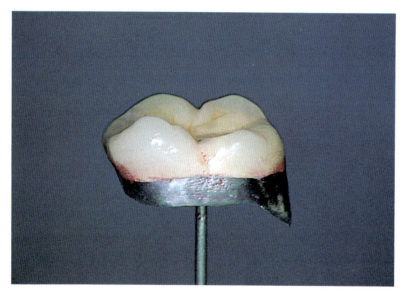

An exposed metal portion similarly affects periodontal health. The metal portion of this crown is porous and therefore cannot be finished smoothly. This shows the importance of a dense, non-porous casting.

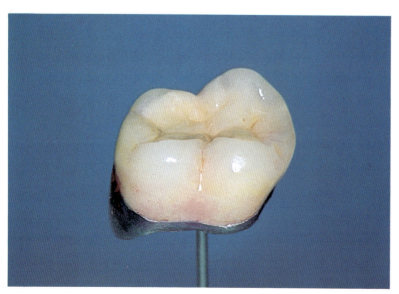

The porcelain crown surface must be given a dense finish through proper condensation of its particles. Although there are many existing condensation methods, the manual skill of the technician ultimately determines the success or failure of the restoration. Careless manipulation of materials creates a coarse surface on the crown. This photograph shows a case in which poor condensation prevented the desired surface smoothness. The combined application of a horn impact mallet and ultra sonic condensation guarantees the desired result. (Refer to Vol. II Chapter 5.) The crowns illustrated on page 40 and page 37 (center) were experimentally placed in the author's mouth for several months to prove that correct restoration of teeth must guarantee self-cleansability.

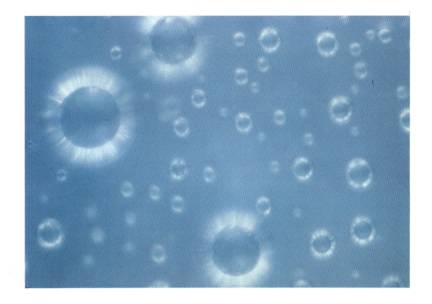

In this case, the layer of glazing and coloring powder has been applied too heavily to compensate for poor condensation. Since those powders contain metal oxides and boric acids, the finished surface presents an impression comparable to moon craters. Boric acid melts at a lower temperature than the firing temperature of the porcelain and thus evaporates.

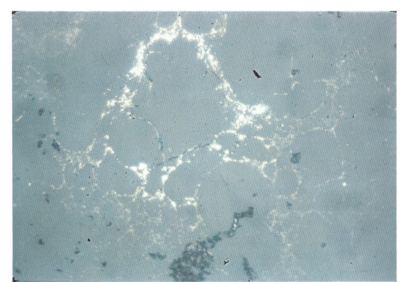

The same magnification of the illustration above, but at a different depth. The difference between the melting temperature of the glazing powder and the firing temperature of the porcelain has caused cracks to occur.

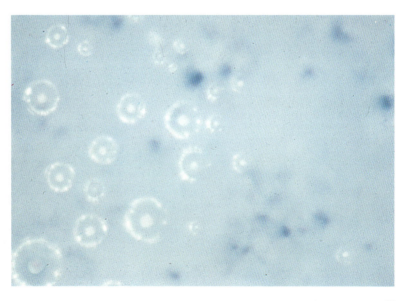

The left side of this illustration shows glazed porcelain, and the right side shows self-glazed porcelain. The contrast is clear enough: on the boundary line, where the layer of glazing powder is thin, we see fewer porosities.

Using glazing powder makes it possible to obtain a somewhat smooth surface, but the best surface quality can be guaranteed only by using self-glazing porcelain.

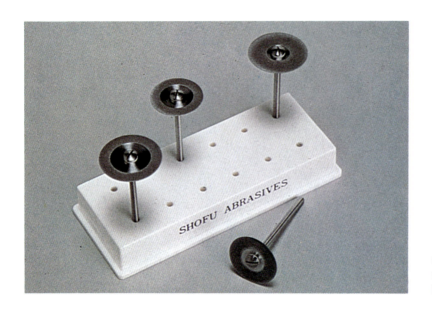

The type of finishing stone or disc used on self-glazing porcelan determines both the smoothness and surface appearance of a restoration after self-glazing is completed.

Surface coarseness of materials and self-glazing

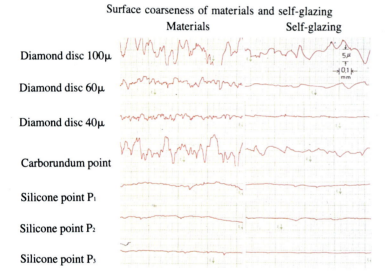

A comparison of the surface coarseness of different materials and of various types of stones and disks (Shofu products) is shown at the top and center.

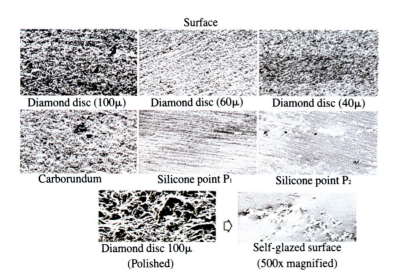

A comparison of micrographs of surface coarseness of stones and disks demonstrates the data illustrated above.

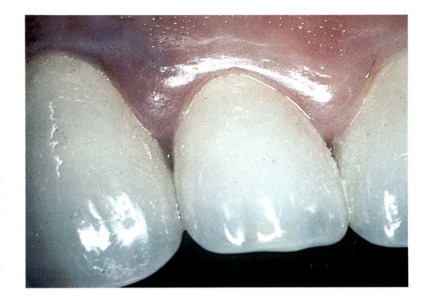

A layer of glazing powder painted on too heavily may flow down to the cervical region of the crown, and the resulting rough porcelain surface will lead to periodontal disease. Shown here are three ceramometal restorations. A thick layer of glazing powder has caused a periodontal problem (photograph courtesy of Dr. G. Straussberg).

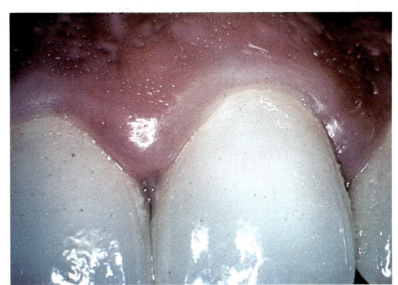

Illustration of a similar case. The small black spots visible on the crown surface may be the result of porosities produced during heavy staining in the laboratory.

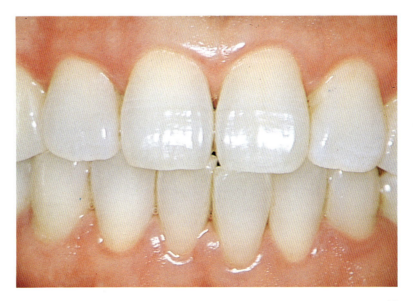

This illustration of a natural dentition shows how smooth texture in the form of concavities and ridges can esthetically improve surface appearance.

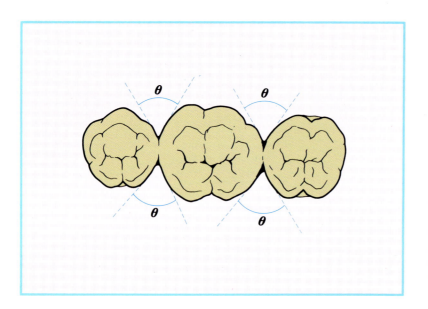

The proximal embrasures are also very important, because if improperly finished, they tend to accumulate dental plaque. Therefore, the embrasure form must always allow for easy cleaning. The proximal embrasure form should be finished with a thin disk (a diamond disk marketed by Shofu Dental Co.).

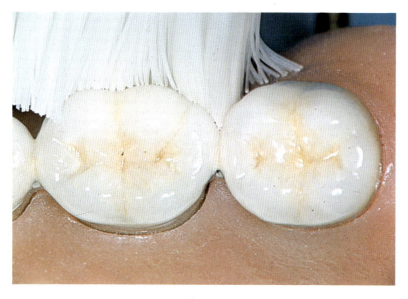

The correctly shaped embrasures allow for easy cleansing.

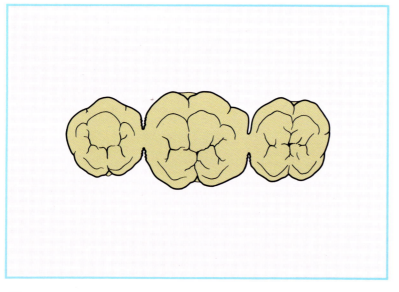

This illustration shows a case of unfavorable proximal embrasure.

2.2 GOALS FOR CROWN DESIGN, USING THE THREE-PLANE CONCEPT

Dental technology is concerned with the design of anatomically correct tooth form; its primary objective is to restore tooth contour in a rational fashion with a minimum expenditure of time. The restoration of the dentition must be carefully planned by establishing goals. Rules governing the contour of teeth are of course directed by concepts of correct dental anatomy and occlusion. Our discussion here will emphasize the concept that the surfaces of the crown portions of any tooth in the dental arch can be visualized as a spatial composition based on three planes.

Through application of this three-plane concept, it is possible to reproduce correct crown form. Similar to the curves of Spee and Wilson and Monson's sphere, these three planes are not always found on the natural tooth. Yet in reference to our dental techniques, this concept is of great importance.

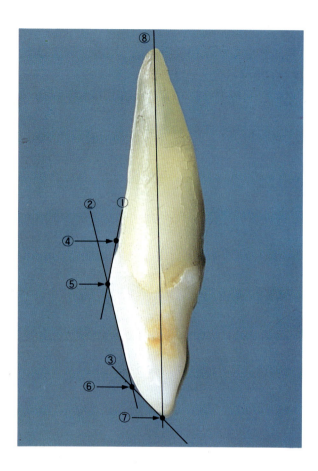

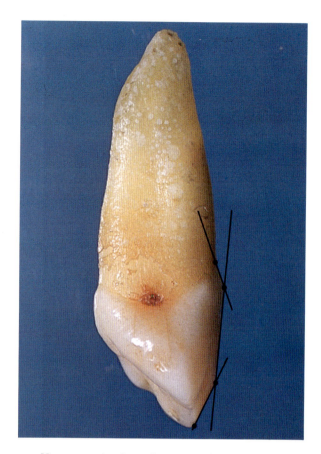

↖ Upon examination of an anterior tooth, we find that its labial side is composed of three planes. Sagittally, it is made up of three of the following planes: the first one running from 1 to 3; the second starting at 2 at the height of contour, and running from 5 to 6; and the 3rd going from the incisal third to the center of the incisal edge. The incisal edge, the interdental papillae, and the root tip are more or less on a straight line.

1) Cervical landmark line on the labial side
1) Cervical landmark line on the lingual side
2) Center landmark line on the labial side
3) Incisal edge landmark line on the lingual side
4) Boundary landmark point on the labial side
5) Cervical landmark point on the labial side
6) Center landmark point on the labial side
7) Incisal edge center landmark point
8) Center line

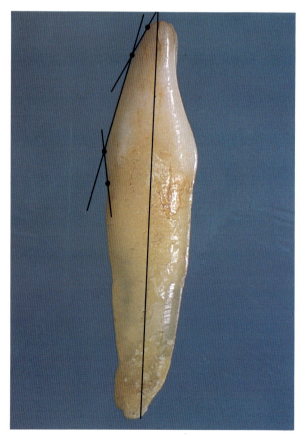

← The labial side of the mandibular central incisor, viewed sagittally. The distance between the two landmark points on the center line is relatively long, and the angle of the center landmark line to the center is small.

↑ Landmark lines and points on the labial side of the maxillary canine.

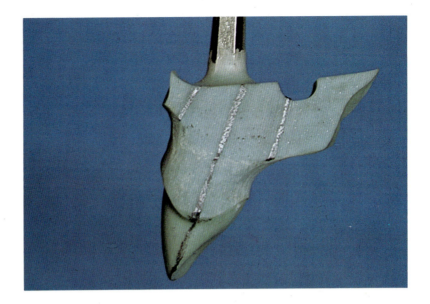

When examined sagittally, the maxillary and mandibular incisors show the center of the incisal edge, the interdental papillae and the root tips in line. During construction of an abutment tooth, the distance between the incisal edge of the tooth and the imaginary line is measured. This helps to determine the direction of the long axis of the tooth.

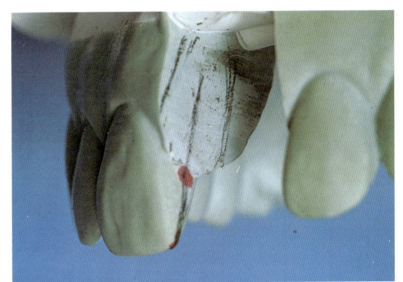

A working cast, on which the center line is marked on the proximal side. Here we see the direction of the long axis.

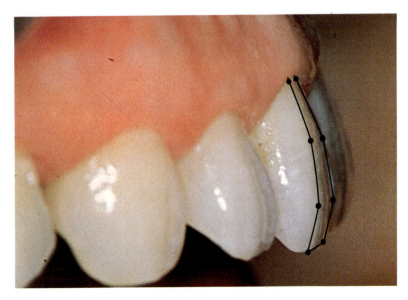

The labial side of the maxillary incisor, viewed proximally from the right. We can observe 3 planes and 2 landmarks indicating the labial curvature.

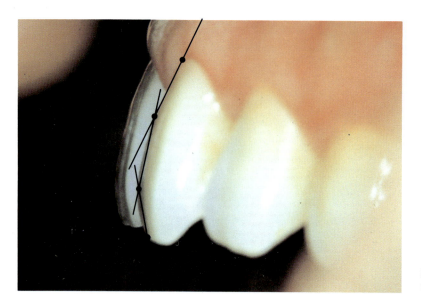

The labial side of the maxillary central incisor, viewed proximally from the left. The three planes can be observed.

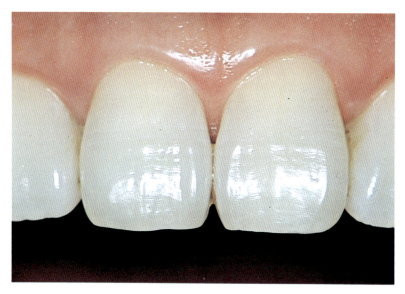

A front view of the above. The shiny surface represents a plane between 2 landmark points on the center line.

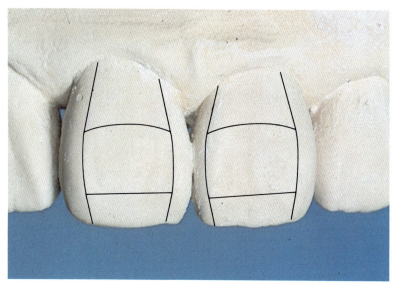

The above maxillary central incisors seen in a cast. The labial side of the maxillary central incisors are shown with their three planes.

The proximal outline of an anterior tooth viewed labially, shown with the three planes.
1) Proximal center line of the cervix, mesial and distal.
2) Proximal center line, mesial and distal center.
3) Proximal marginal line, mesial and distal.
4) Proximal landmark point, mesial and distal boundary.
5) Proximal center cervical point, mesial and distal cervix line.
6) Proximal center point, mesial and distal center point.
7) Mesial and distal line angle point.

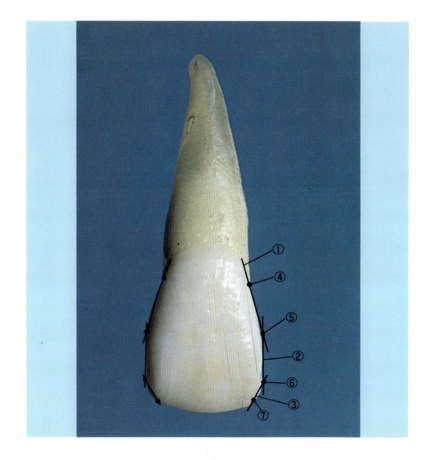

The proximal cervical line is a straight line extending continuously to the root and the proximal center lines, constituting an interproximal contact area. The lengths and angles of these two landmark lines have much to do with the proper function of the teeth. On the other hand, the proximal marginal ridge line is important in esthetics and the individuality of the patient. If various landmark lines were set up as indicated by the red lines, the crown form would be functionally and esthetically incorrect.

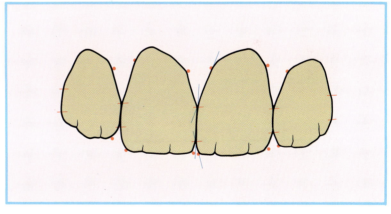

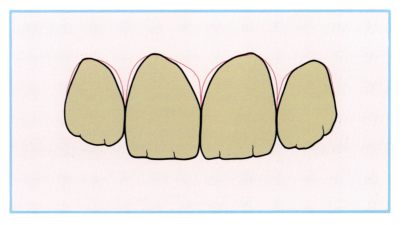

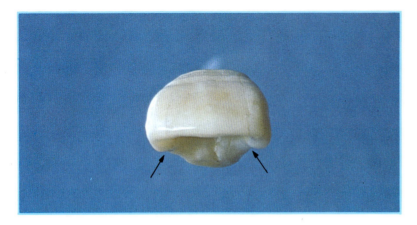

The maxillary central incisor viewed incisally. Two of the three planes constituting the labial side can be seen, as are certain characteristics on the lingual side, including the mesial and distal marginal ridges, the lingual fossa, the cingulum and spillways. (as indicated by arrows)

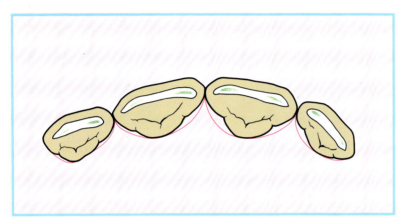

When anterior teeth are overcontoured, gingival tissues are compromised. The food bolus can not find proper spillways, leading to unsatisfactory self-cleansibility.

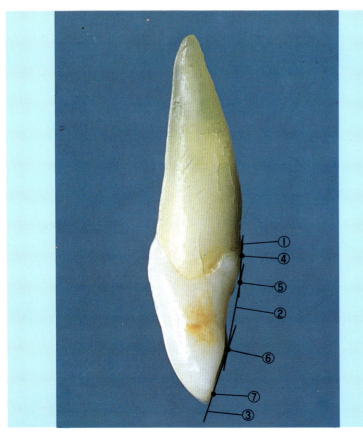

The lingual surface of the anterior teeth, viewed sagittally, is also made up of three planes.

    1) Cervical line on the lingual side
    2) Center line on the lingual side
    3) Incisal edge line on the lingual side
    4) Lingual CE Junction point
    5) Cingulum point
    6) Lingual center point
    7) Incisal edge point on the lingual side

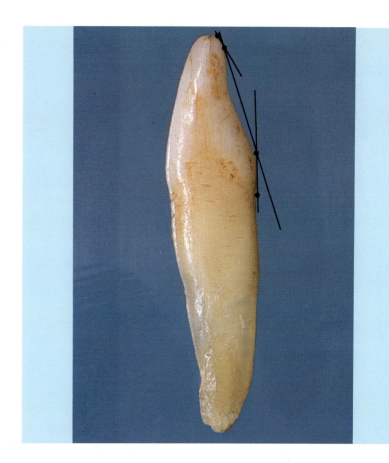

The mandibular central incisor viewed sagittally. As in the above case, we note three landmark lines and four landmark points.

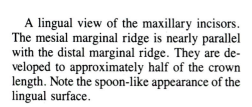

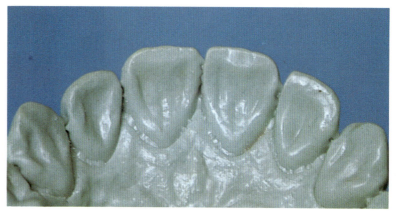

A lingual view of the maxillary incisors. The mesial marginal ridge is nearly parallel with the distal marginal ridge. They are developed to approximately half of the crown length. Note the spoon-like appearance of the lingual surface.

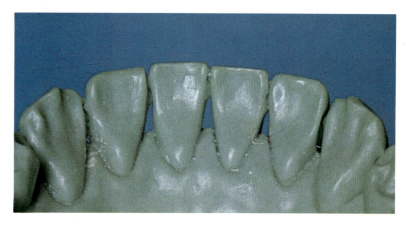

A lingual view of the mandibular central incisors. When compared with the maxillary incisors, the mandibular incisors shows neither well-developed marginal ridges nor a lingual fossa. A depression on the lingual side, common in both the maxillary and mandibular anteriors, is characteristic of the human anterior teeth.

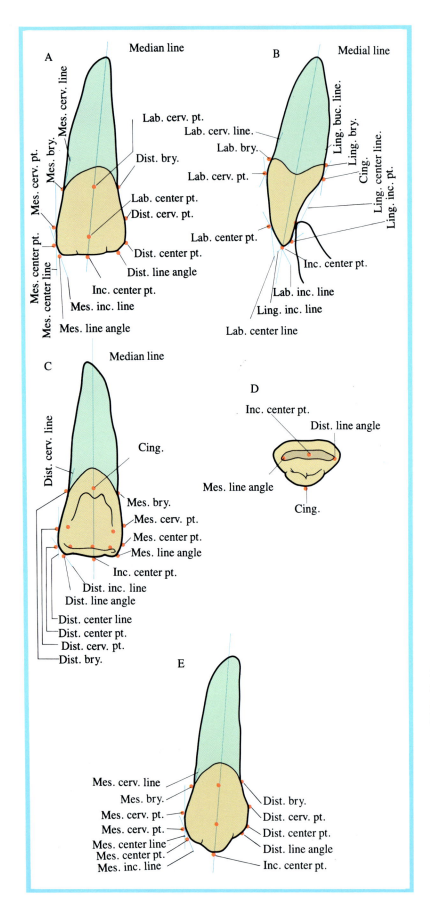

A

Median line

Mes. cerv. line
Mes. bry.
Mes. cerv. pt.
Mes. cerv. pt.
Mes. center pt.
Mes. center line
Mes. center line
Mes. inc. line
Mes. line angle

Lab. cerv. pt.
Lab. cerv. line.
Lab. bry.
Dist. bry.
Lab. center pt.
Dist. cerv. pt.
Lab. center pt.
Dist. center pt.
Dist. line angle
Inc. center pt.

B

Medial line

Ling. buc. line.
Ling. bry.
Ling. center line.
Cing.
Ling. center line.
Ling. inc. pt.

Lab. cerv. line.
Lab. bry.
Lab. cerv. pt.
Lab. center pt.

Inc. center pt.
Lab. inc. line
Ling. inc. line
Lab. center line

C

Median line

Dist. cerv. line

Cing.

Mes. bry.
Mes. cerv. pt.
Mes. center pt.
Mes. line angle
Inc. center pt.
Dist. inc. line
Dist. line angle
Dist. center line
Dist. center pt.
Dist. cerv. pt.
Dist. bry.

D

Inc. center pt.
Dist. line angle
Mes. line angle
Cing.

E

Mes. cerv. line
Mes. bry.
Mes. cerv. pt.
Mes. cerv. pt.
Mes. center line
Mes. center pt.
Mes. inc. line

Dist. bry.
Dist. cerv. pt.
Dist. center pt.
Dist. line angle
Inc. center pt.

Boundary = bry.
Buccal = buc.
Cervical = cerv.
Cingulum = cing.
Distal = dist.
Incisal = inc.
Lingual = ling.
Mesial = mes.
Point = pt.

When planning the construction of the functional crown form, the various landmarks, lines, and ridges provide us with guidelines for the procedural steps of our project.

A. Landmark lines and points on the maxillary incisor, labial view.
B. Landmark lines and points on the maxillary incisor, sagittal view.
C. Landmark lines and points on the maxillary incisor, lingual view
D. Landmark lines and points on the maxillary incisor, incisal view.
E. Landmark lines and points on the maxillary canine, labial view.

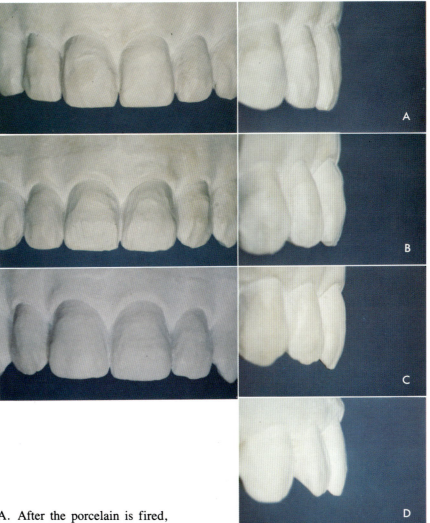

Illustration A. After the porcelain is fired, the restoraton is adjusted initially with the soft gingiva model as a guide. An impression of this is transferred to a plaster model. Three planes can be envisioned when viewed from the proximal direction, but since the incisal edge is angulated incorrectly, these restorations lack a natural appearance. The labial landmark lines are insufficient.

Illustration B. The above porcelain crowns are modified and an impression of the maxillary cast poured in model plaster. In this modification, efforts are made to create a smooth transition to the root as determined by the soft gingiva model; harmony with the gingival tissues and correct proximal embrasures based on the three-plane concept are the ultimate goal here.

Illustration C. The angles are provided by the mesiodistal labial plane from a proximal direction with rugae transversely running on the labial surface. A stone is used in this final finishing process.

Illustration D. A cast of a patient's natural teeth. In order to obtain a close similarity to the natural tooth, the center point of the incisal edge needs to be placed on its center line in reference to our three basic planes. Once the project is properly planned, even a beginner can fabricate a fully functional and esthetically pleasing porcelain restoration.

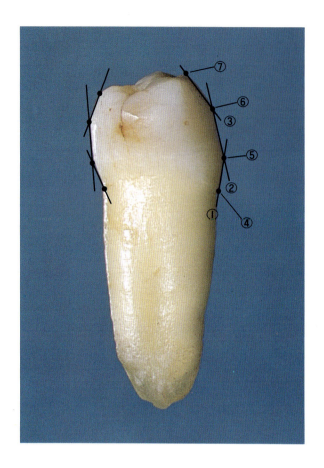

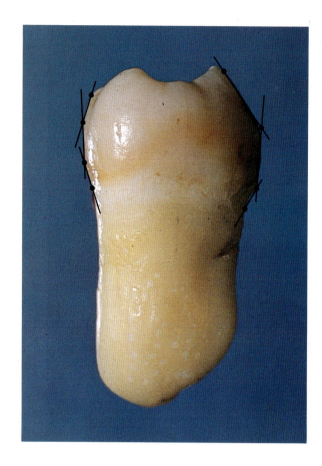

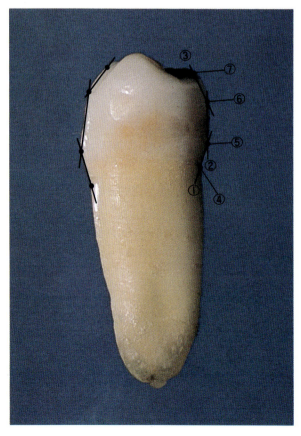

← Left: The buccolingual surface of a premolar consists again of three planes. The planes and landmark points are as follows:

1) Buccal cervical line
2) Buccal center line
3) Buccal cusp line
4) Buccal boundary point
5) Buccal center cervical point
6) Buccal center point
7) Buccal cusp tip point

← The lingual plane of a premolar has the same combination of landmark lines and points.

1) Lingual cervical line
2) Lingual center line
3) Lingual cusp line
4) Lingual boundary point
5) Lingual center cervical point
6) Lingual center point
7) Lingual cusp tip point

↑ The landmark lines and points on a molar.

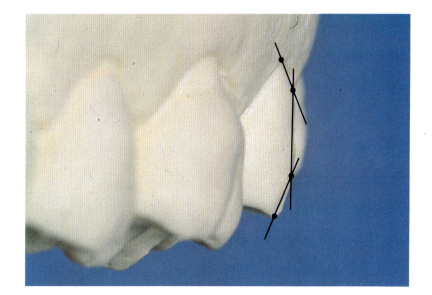

The buccal planes of the maxillary molars are organized in similar manner.

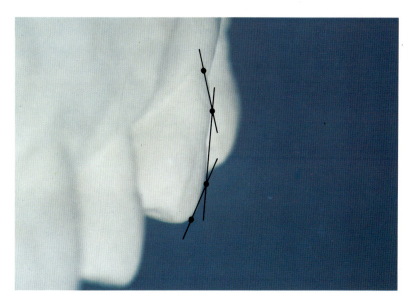

The buccal planes of the maxillary first molar are organized similarly.

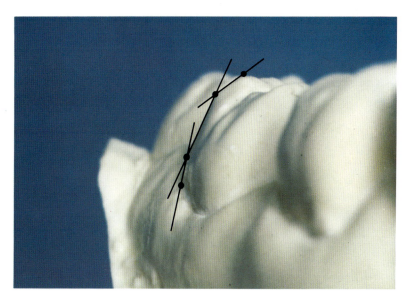

The same 3-plane concept is used for the buccal surfaces of the mandibular molars.

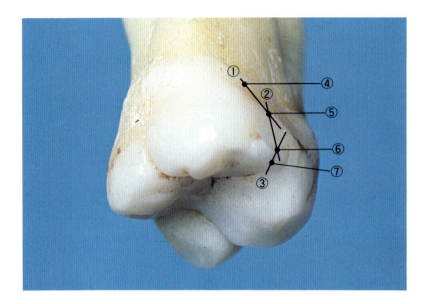

The proximal surface of the molar is again established by three planes.

1) Proximal cervical line, mesial and distal.
2) Proximal center line, mesial and distal center.
3) Proximal marginal ridge line, mesial and distal.
4) Proximal boundary point, mesial and distal.
5) Proximal center cervical point, mesial and distal.
6) Proximal center point, mesial and distal.
7) Mesial and distal line angle point.

The proximal cervical line is a straight line in continuous transition to the root and the proximal center line, forming a contact area between proximal surfaces.

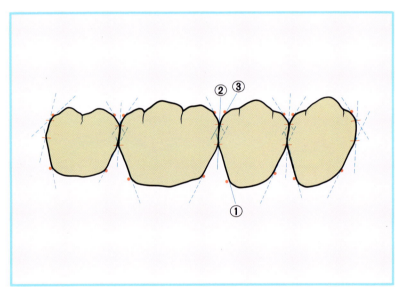

The angle and distance of the proximal cusp line greatly influence the function, esthetics, and individuality of a restoration. On the other hand, the proximal cervical line and proximal center line are linked only to function.

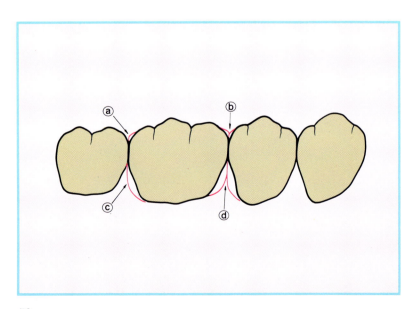

If the lines constituting the proximal molar surface are placed as indicated in red, severe irritation of the gingival tissues results.
a. Food impaction at the embrasures is likely to occur, preventing proper cleansing in those areas.
b. The gingiva is placed under pressure, also resulting in lack of self-cleansability.

Boundary = bry.
Buccal = buc.
Cervical = cerv.
Distal = dist.
Lingual = ling.
Mesial = mes.
Point = pt.

A

Dist. line angle
Dist. center pt.
Dist. cerv. pt.
Dist. bry.
Buc. cerv. pt.

Buc. cusp tip pt.
Mes. cusp line
Mes. line angle
Mes. center pt.
Mes. cerv. pt.
Mes. center line
Mes. bry.
Mes. cerv. line

B

Buc. center line
Buc. center pt.

Buc. cerv. pt.
Buc. bry.
Buc. cerv. line.

Buc. cusp line
Buc. cusp tip pt.
Ling. cusp line
Ling. cusp tip pt.
Ling. center pt.

Ling. cerv. pt.
Ling. center line
Ling. bry.
Ling. cerv. line

C

Ling. cusp tip pt.
Mes. line angle
Mes. center pt.
Mes. cerv. pt.
Mes. bry.

Buc. cusp tip pt.
Dist. cusp line
Dist. line angle
Dist. center pt.
Dist. cerv. line
Dist. center line
Dist. bry.
Ling. cerv. pt.
Dist. cerv. line

D

Mes. line angle
Marg. ridge pt.

Buc. cerv. pt.
Buc. cusp tip pt.
Dist. line angle
Ling. cusp pt.
Ling. cerv. pt.

Landmark lines and points for the mandibular premolar are indicated. The basic rules also apply to the maxillary premolar.
  A. Respective lines and points on the buccal plane.
  B. Respective lines and points on the sagittal plane.
  C. Respective lines and points on the lingual plane.
  D. Respective lines and points on the occlusal surface.

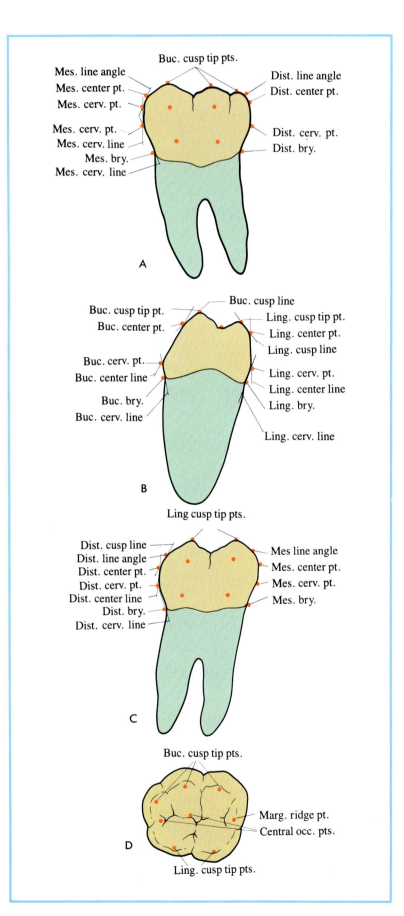

A

Buc. cusp tip pts.

Mes. line angle
Mes. center pt.
Mes. cerv. pt.

Dist. line angle
Dist. center pt.

Mes. cerv. pt.
Mes. cerv. line
Mes. bry.
Mes. cerv. line

Dist. cerv. pt.
Dist. bry.

B

Buc. cusp line

Buc. cusp tip pt.
Buc. center pt.

Ling. cusp tip pt.
Ling. center pt.
Ling. cusp line

Buc. cerv. pt.
Buc. center line

Ling. cerv. pt.
Ling. center line
Ling. bry.

Buc. bry.
Buc. cerv. line

Ling. cerv. line

C

Ling cusp tip pts.

Dist. cusp line
Dist. line angle
Dist. center pt.
Dist. cerv. pt.
Dist. center line
Dist. bry.
Dist. cerv. line

Mes line angle
Mes. center pt.
Mes. cerv. pt.
Mes. bry.

D

Buc. cusp tip pts.

Marg. ridge pt.
Central occ. pts.

Ling. cusp tip pts.

Boundary = bry.
Buccal = buc.
Cervical = cerv.
Distal = dist.
Incisal = inc.
Lingual = ling.
Marginal = marg.
Mesial = mes.
Occlusal = occ.
Point = pt.

Landmark lines and points for the mandibular molar are indicated. The principles are also applicable to the maxillary molar.

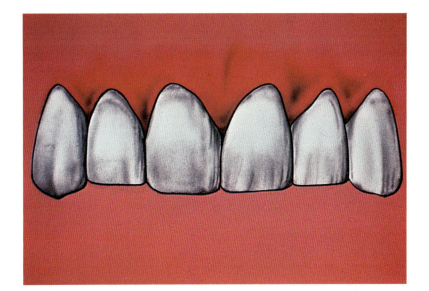

According to Dr. R.S. Stein, the cervical gingival line seen from the labial side of the maxillary anteriors and surrounded by healthy gingiva is not semilunar, but forms a zonal triangle with the tips moved distally.

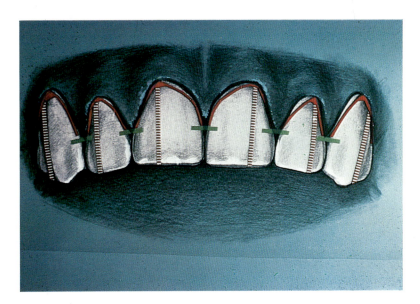

The tip of this zonal triangle is said to be in a position of ⅓ of the crown distally. This point should be kept in mind during construction of the wax pattern.

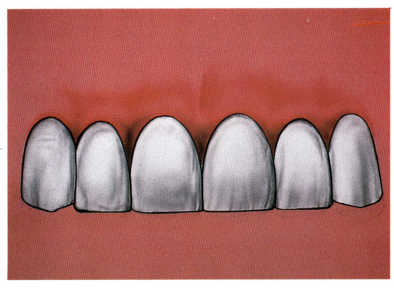

When the gingiva is not healthy, the cervical gingival line often presents a semilunar appearance (photographs courtesy of Dr. R.S. Stein).

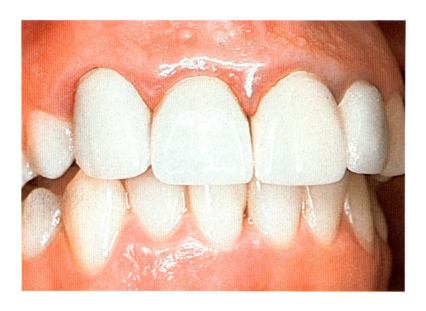

Restorations after 6 years (a collaboration with Dr. R.S. Stein).

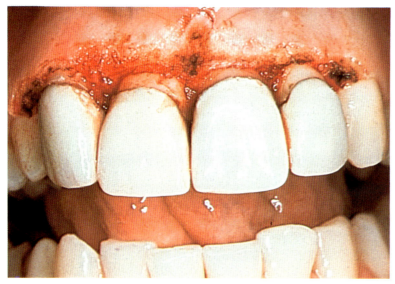

A preoperative view of a case treatment planned for ceramometal restorations, where the maxillary 6 anteriors are to be treated periodontally and prosthodontically (photograph courtesy of Dr. R.S. Stein).

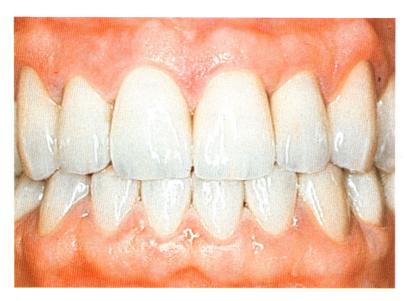

The entire maxillary and mandibular reconstruction completed by the author for Dr. S. Wagman (after several years). See also Vol. II, Ch. 9.

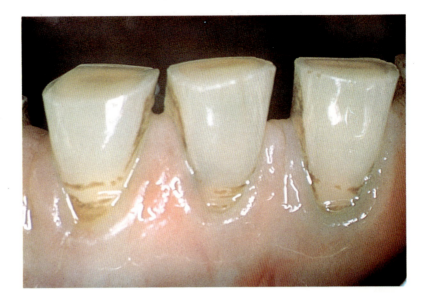

Preoperative view

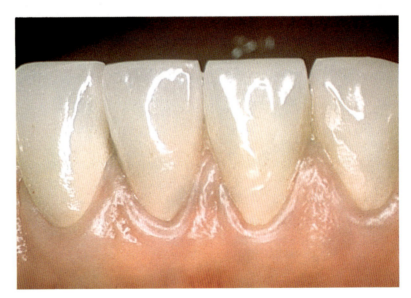

Postoperative view after 9 years (photograph courtesy of Dr. S. Wagman).

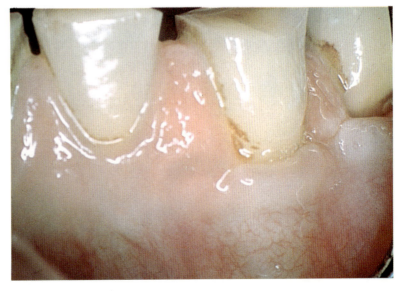

Preoperative view of the same case — lateral view (photograph courtesy of Dr. S. Wagman).

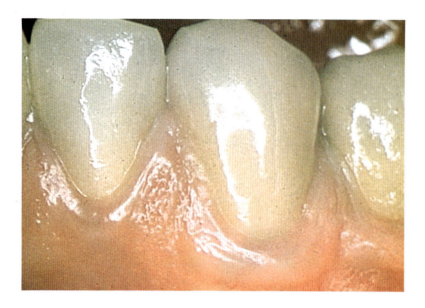

Postoperative view of the previous case after 6 years (photograph courtesy of Dr. S. Wagman).

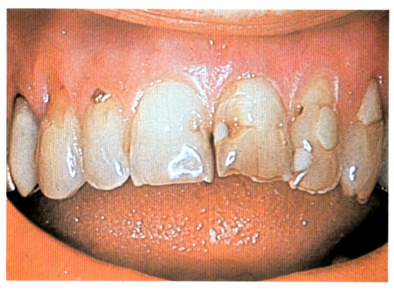

Preoperative view of another case.

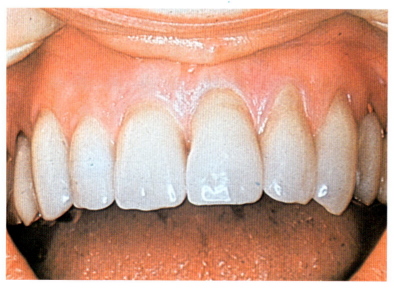

Postoperative view of the same case (both photographs courtesy of Dr. R.S. Stein).

2.3 CONTOUR GUIDELINES AND THE SOFT GINGIVA MODEL

In the process of restoring tooth form, in order to achieve total balance, the following considerations are essential: the maintenance of gingival health; the restoration of masticatory, phonetic, and esthetic function; and the requirement of strength. Primary consideration, however, must be given to maintenance of gingival health.

The construction of crowns and fixed partial dentures must also focus on the functional relationship of the teeth; on the periodontal apparatus (including the alveolar bone); and on the functions of the lips, cheeks, and tongue. That portion of the fired restoration which does not come into contact with the tongue should be finished to the highest degree of smoothness, since deposition of calculus can not be prevented by tongue movement. For better self-cleansability of the restoration, a large contact area is desirable on the buccal side between the buccinator muscle and the gingiva and crown surface. It is important to have the buccinator contact the lateral side of the crown and the gingival surfaces as evenly as possible.

Contour is closely linked to the health of the gingival tissues. When a margin is placed subgingivally, its relation to the abutment teeth and the state of the gingival tissues must be closely observed. When a restoration shows correct gingival contour, it is somewhat difficult to observe the effect of muscular movement and function in that area, but by establishing a standardized step by step procedure we can learn the muscular movement and function involved.

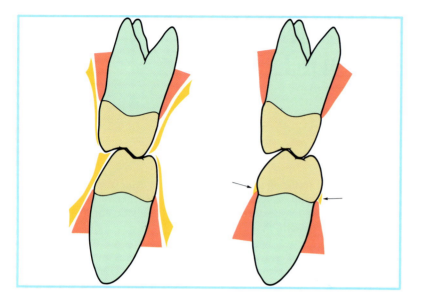

A correctly contoured crown compatible with the gingival tissues will prevent deposition of plaque through proper flow of the food bolus. Proper flow of the food bolus favorably stimulates the gingiva and thus contributes to its health. When a crown is over-contoured, the result is an unfavorable flow of food particles. For an examination of crown contour, the fabrication of a plaster cast is helpful. A better method for the study of the soft tissues is the transfer of the gingival portion onto a soft material, thus providing a tactile knowledge of the state of the soft tissues. This replacement of the gingival portion with a soft material has been advocated by Dr. Pinkas.

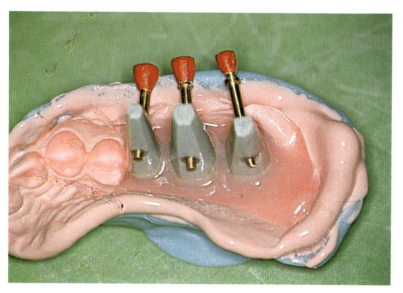

Currently, rubber impression materials are available, in addition to soft resin denture products, as shown in this illustration.

ADVANTAGES OF THE SOFT GINGIVA MODEL

1. It facilitates recognition of the gingiva's condition.
   a. A margin can be determined with the naked eye.
   b. Contour guidelines can be obtained on the labial, buccal, and lingual surfaces.
   c. It provides a clear view of the height and contour of the papillae.
2. The direction of the root can be examined.
   a. In reference to the relationship between cusps and root.
   b. To facilitate the obtainment of biological and functional transition form between root and crown contour.

As this illustration shows, the objective of the soft gingiva model is to obtain proper crown contour.

On a well contoured natural tooth surrounded by healthy gingiva, the labiolingual contour lines of the crown are either identical with a straight line contacting the gingiva or are placed within the boundary. This straight line contacting the gingiva is referred to as a buccal, labial, or lingual contour line.

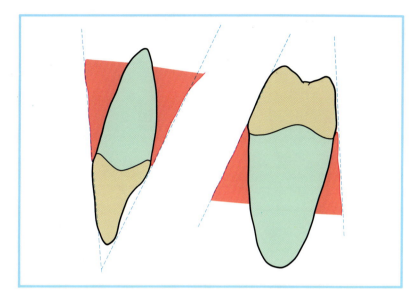

Of the three landmark lines forming the anterior labial and lingual surfaces, the cervical line coincides with the inner surface of the gingiva while the center line is identical with the outer surface of the gingiva. By using a soft gingiva model, we can obtain the three labial-cervical, lingual-cervical and lingual-incisal edge points, as indicated in (1), (2), and (3). Moreover, from the soft gingival model, the position of the interdental papilla (4) can be derived. This is a line connecting the abutment with it (5), the incisal edge center point (6), the labial incisal edge line (7), and the lingual incisal edge line (8) for phonetic and esthetic considerations.

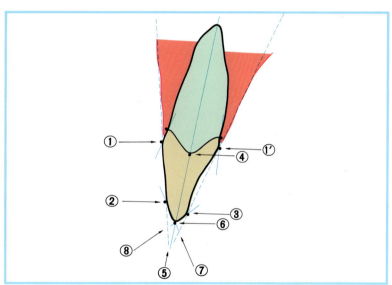

Of the three lines that constitute the buccal and lingual surfaces of the molar crown, the cervical line coincides with the inner wall of the gingiva, as with the anterior teeth. The center line is nearly identical with the contour guideline. We can also derive from the soft gingival model the buccolabial and buccolingual cervical point (1) and (1'), and the center points (2) and (3). On the molars, the distance between the cusp tips accounts for about 55-60% of the buccolingual maximum width. Here the buccal occlusal (4), the lingual occlusal (5), and the buccal and lingual cusp tip points (6) and (6') are established in reference to the teeth of the opposing arch.

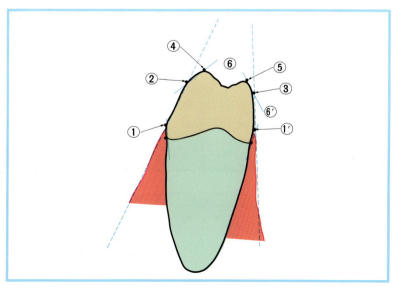

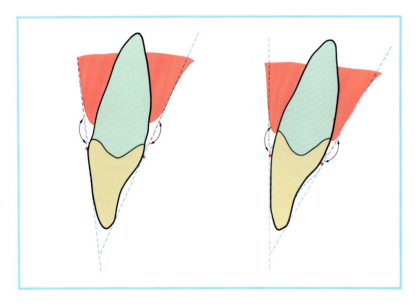

In the case of gingival recession, reproduction of the exposed root guarantees a harmonious crown contour without changing the positions of the labial cervical and cingulum points. When root contour remains unmodified, it is necessary to position these two points further within the contour guidelines.

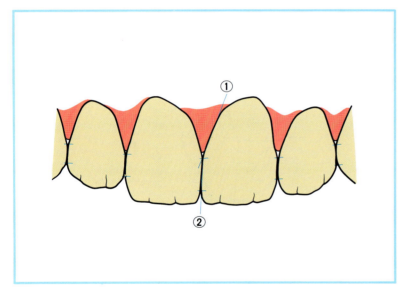

Since the soft gingiva model indicates the height and contour of the interdental papilla, the contact area and its lower limit is shown by the proximal cervical line (1). In any case, pressure on the gingiva must be avoided at all costs. The boundary center line (2) is determined by taking into account the triangular contour of the interdental papilla, individual differences in crown form, and harmony with facial features.

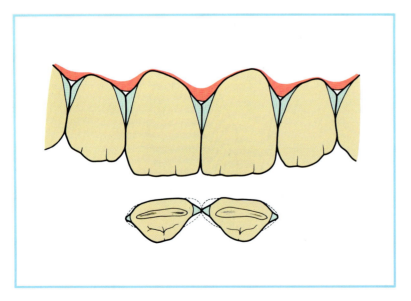

In the case of gingival atrophy, where the interdental papilla has become flat, the proximal contour must be established by three planes (viewed from the front). In anterior restorations, the interdental papilla area is sometimes filled in for esthetic reasons. In such a situation, contact is kept light in the center of the labiolingual surface and becomes shallower apically. Thus, oral hygiene is facilitated, phonetics are improved, and the appearance of the restoration is esthetically pleasing.

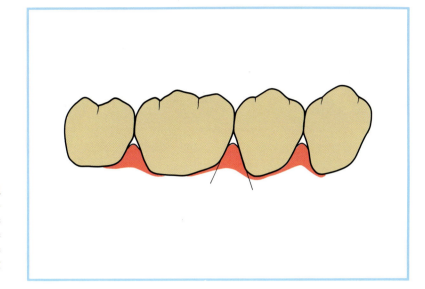

The proximal molar contour is constructed in three planes, as seen from the lateral aspect. Since the most important role of the molar is its function, the contact area must be contoured so as not to exert pressure on the gingiva, while at the same time providing sufficient room for oral hygiene.

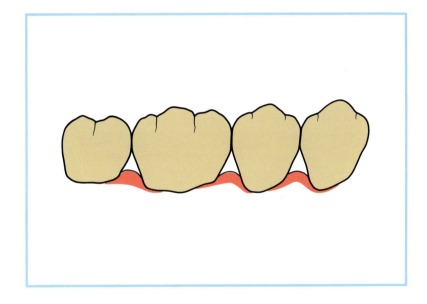

When treating a molar with an atrophied interdental papilla, sufficient embrasure width for self-cleansing must be provided; here the problems of phonetics and esthetics are secondary.

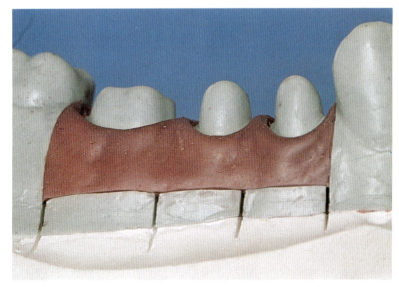

The direction of the root can be determined from the soft gingiva model and that direction then used to help position the cusps properly. Thus, information on the biological and functional transition of the crown to the root surface is also available.

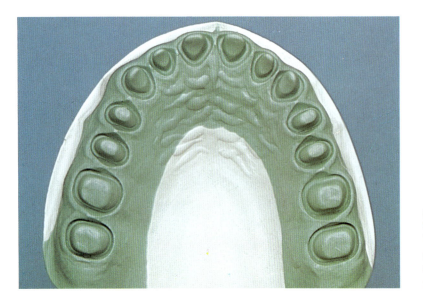

The fabricaton of the soft gingiva model.

Several methods of fabricating a soft gingiva model exist; our discussion involves one that can be used for multiple restorations. This model is prepared before the dies are separated and trimmed. The photograph shows a maxillary soft gingiva model before separation and trimming of the dies.

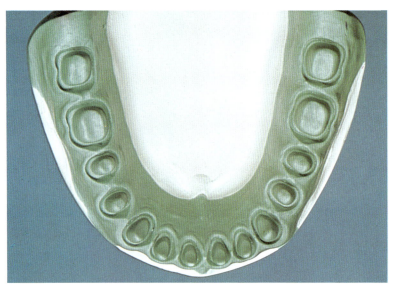

This figure shows a mandibular soft gingiva model.

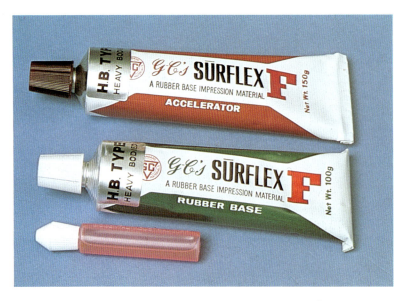

The material used for this type of model must be distortion-free and guarantee high dimensional stability. The pigmentation of the material is also important. In this case, an impression was made with polysulfide rubber impression material and silicone impression material was used for the gingival portion.

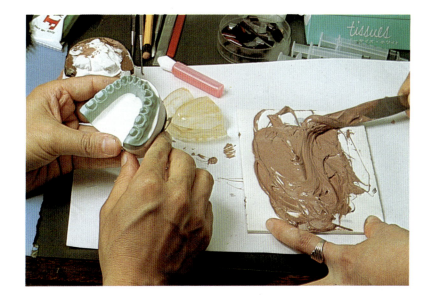

A polysulfide rubber impression material is used here, having been mixed according to the manufacturer's instructions.

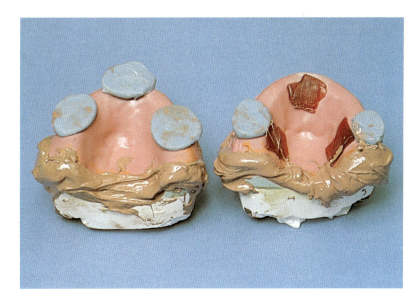

The maxillary and mandibular impressions are made with Polysulfide. When using elastomeric impression materials, it is important to use a custom tray. Polymer resin pads as holding devices for the impression trays will ease the removal of the set impression.

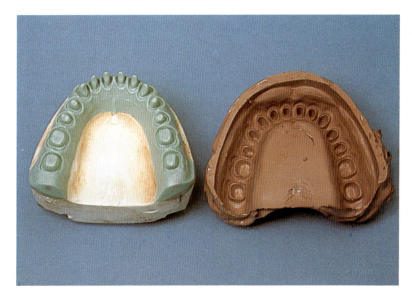

When making the final impression, it is important that the gingival contour be accurately registered throughout the dental arch.

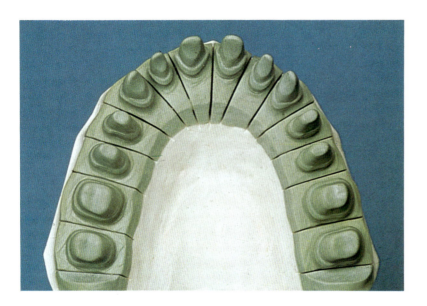

A maxillary working cast in which die separation and trimming have been completed.

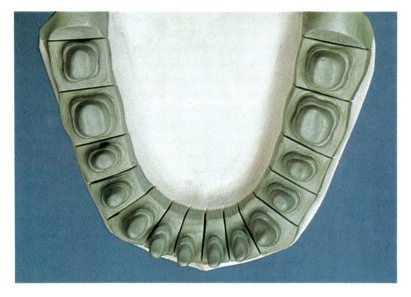

A mandibular working model.

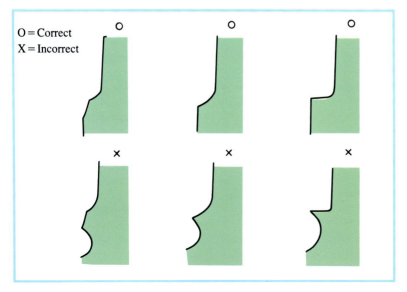

O = Correct
X = Incorrect

When trimming the margin, the following must be observed:
1. The margin must be clearly visible from the outside.
2. The marginal line should be hard enough not to easily break down.
3. The trimming beneath the margin must be parallel both mesiodistally and labiolingually.

Therefore, as illustrated, cutting deeply beneath the margin must be avoided.

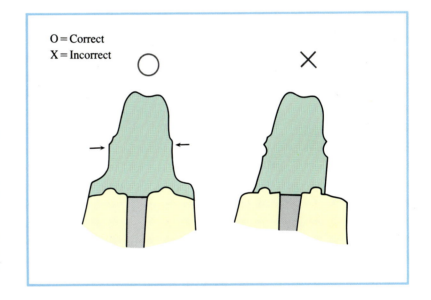

Cutting the margin concave will result in the following disadvantages:
1. An instrument is apt to injure the margin during trimming
2. During waxing, some of the wax may find its way into the margin
3. The margin of a model may be fractured by trying the crown on the die after casting

In a tooth preparation with little taper, trimming part of the margin (indicated by arrow) is inevitable. But a parallel relationship of the mesio-distal and buccolingual surfaces should be gradually maintained. A portion corresponding to the cingulum must be spaced wide enough to effect harmony with the gingiva; this, in turn, will prevent rotation. A lock model of sufficient strength is recommended here; a rotatory prevention device of the semiround type is best prepared on a smooth surface. The illustration on the right side shows incorrect management of such a situation.

O = Correct
X = Incorrect

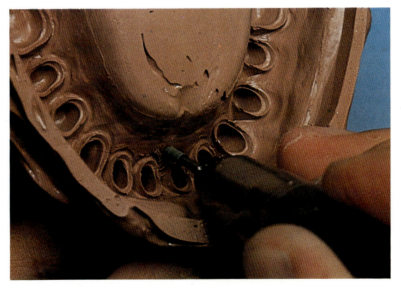

A hole is made on the lingual side of the impression, into which silicone is poured to serve as soft gingiva. Two holes are also made on the right and left posterior areas for the injection and ejection of the impression material.

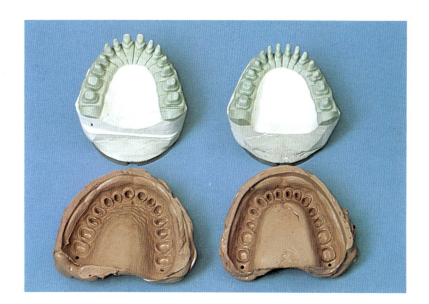

Maxillary and mandibular models on which die separation and trimming have been completed. (Note: holes for injection and ejection of the impression material.)

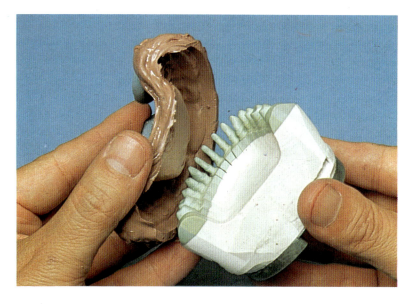

The impression is returned to a prepared working cast. Space obtained by trimming the polysulfide will subsequently be filled with silicone impression material.

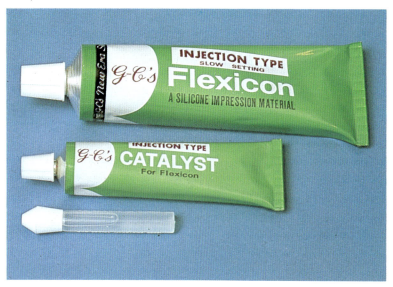

A type of silicone impression material used as soft gingiva material. It must be given a color similar to the natural gingiva of the patient.

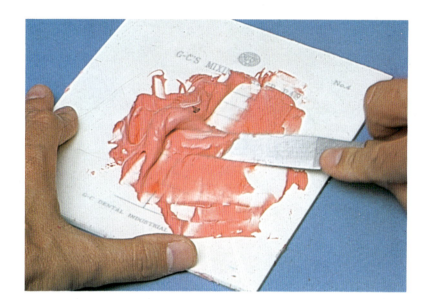

The silicone impression material is mixed.

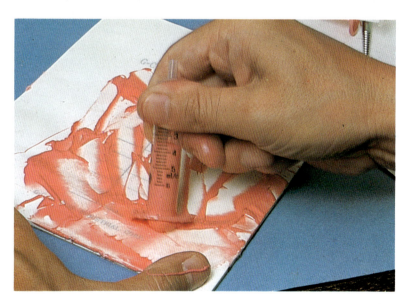

The material is placed in a syringe.

The impression material is injected under pressure into previously formed holes until the excess material is ejected from other holes. If material is ejected from one hole only, the procedure is kept up until material penetrates to the other hole.

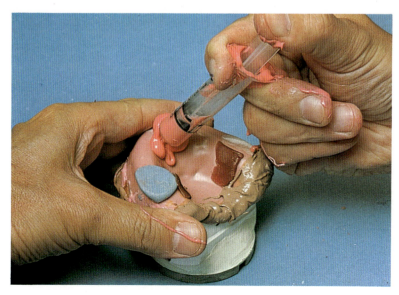

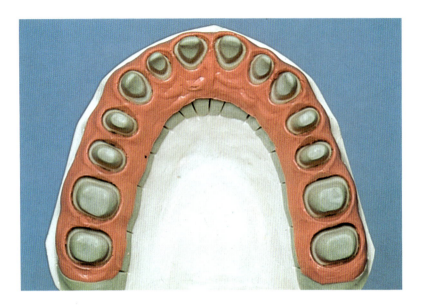

A completed maxillary soft gingiva model. It is subsequently separated into individual dies and mounted on an articulator. When a silicone material is used for model duplication, polysulfide rubber is used as soft gingiva material.

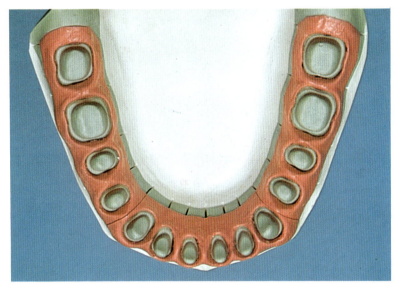

A finished mandibular soft gingiva model.

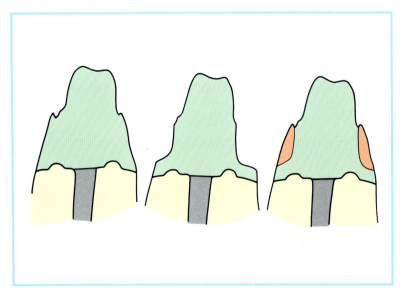

A schematic illustration showing the relationship between the trimmed dies, gingival region, and soft gingiva.

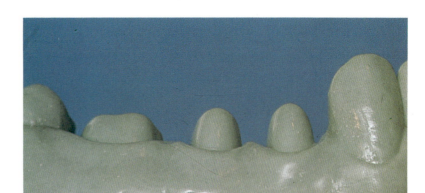

Fabrication of the soft gingiva model (2).

Another illustration of fabricaton of the soft gingiva model. This is a convenient method particularly adapted to manufacturing a single crown or bridge. The model is shown prior to separation and trimming of the dies.

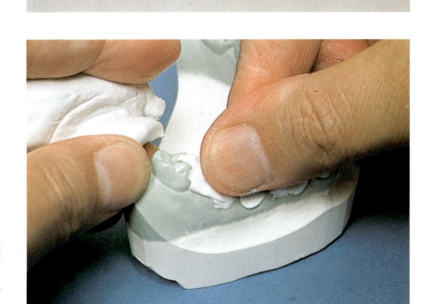

Heavy putty-type silicone impression material is used for an impression of the adjacent teeth and surrounding tissues. The cervical and gingival regions in particular require application of sufficient pressure in order to adapt the material well.

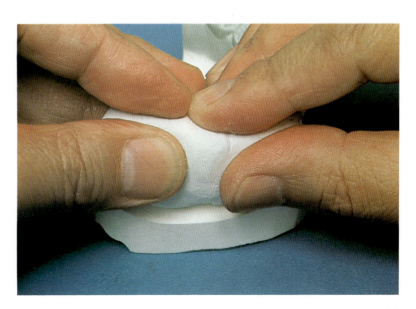

Uniform pressure is applied to the impression material until it has firmly set.

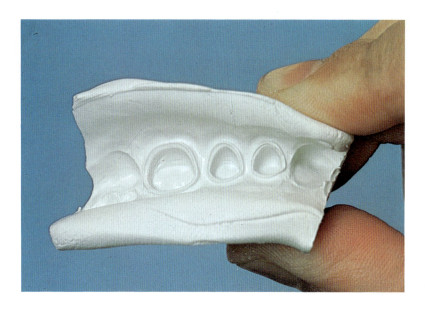

The set impression.

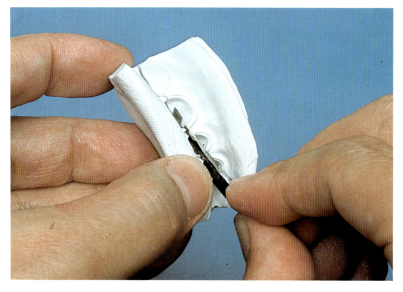

The above impression is separated buccolingually.

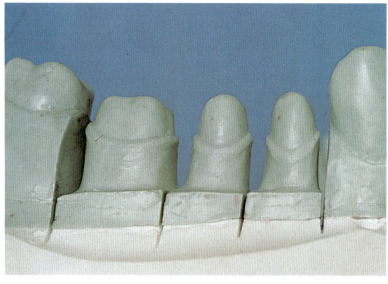

After the separation and trimming of the dies, the impression is prepared for the working model. The trimmed part wll be transferred as soft gingiva.

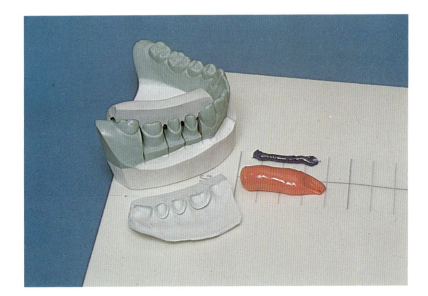

Putty slicone material is used in connection with rubber base impression material, so that the latter will not adhere to the former.

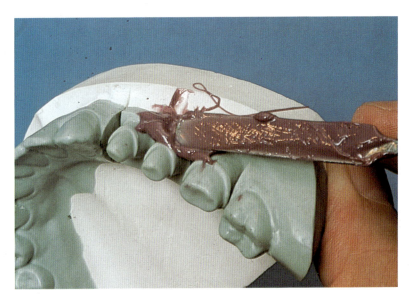

The material is added onto the buccolingual surface exceeding the amount of the trimmed material.

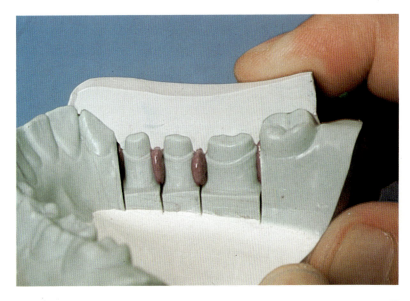

The buccal portion of the previously prepared putty slicone impression is firmly fitted onto the buccal side of the model. Thus the impression material can be pressed into the area with sufficient force so that its excess penetrates through the proximal areas.

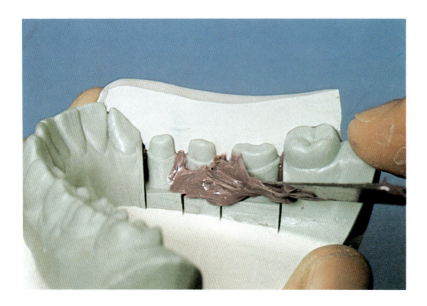

In our next step, the material is added onto the lingual surface.

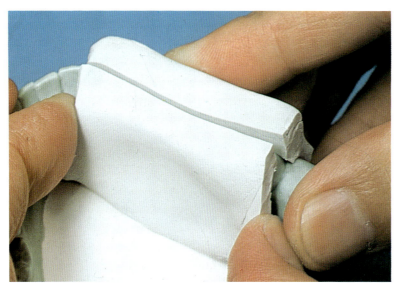

The lingual portion of the putty silicone must be fitted exactly over the impression.

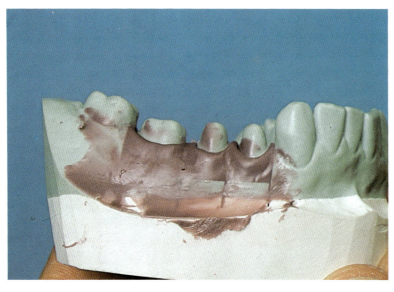

After the material has set, the buccolingual side of the putty silicone impression is removed. As indicated in this illustration, the impression material shows up as a thin layer.

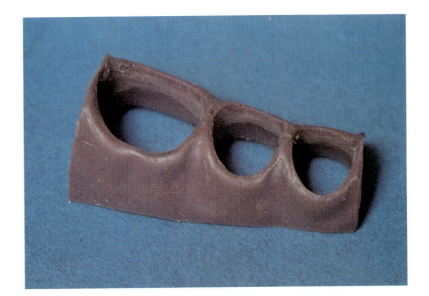

The excess material is cut off to finish the soft gingiva.

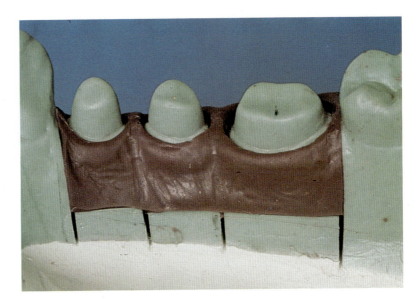

The soft gingiva is then used as material for the soft gingiva model. Since this type of impression material cannot simulate the natural gingival appearance, this does present some clinical inconvenience.

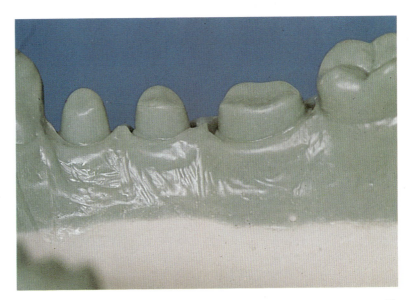

A model before separation and trimming of the dies. Notice that the gingiva is well reproduced in the soft gingival model shown above.

3

FABRICATION OF THE WAX PATTERN (SKELETAL TECHNIQUE)

As described in the previous section, the crown surface contour is basically made up of three planes. In order to arrive at an anatomically correct wax pattern, the spatial surfaces of the crown must be established. To carry out a large scale ceramometal restoration, it is essential to draw a three-dimensional design as a guideline for the final contour. The skeletal technique provides a systematic approach for the waxing procedures. Functional landmarks are waxed up in preparation for the ceramometal restoration.

The discussion here will focus on the restoration of the maxillary and mandibular anterior teeth and the mandibular molars, using the skeletal technique for the three-dimensional waxing procedure. Those concepts are directly applicable to wax patterns for the complete cast and ceramometal crown. Reference is also made to the restoration of one molar in proximal contact with adjacent teeth. Since crown preparation should never be a product of trial and error, it must be based on sound planning. Proper planning guarantees an unfailing restoration based on sound functional and esthetic principals.

3.1 PLANNING THE CROWN CONSTRUCTION: OBJECTIVES

In large scale restorations of one or more maxillary or mandibular quadrants with ceramometal castings, all aspects of occlusion must be considered. When building up porcelain on a cast metal structure that has been modified and heat-treated, the movements of the condyles (posterior guidance), anterior guidance, occlusal surfaces, positioning of the molar cusp tips, and the angles of their inclined planes and cusp ridges must be taken into consideration. Only an understanding of those factors will guarantee successful porcelain restoration. We must be able to predict the final shape of the restoration.

Without a detailed plan and an exact scale drawing of the design, we cannot expect a well-executed restoration. With well-planned designs and specific goals in mind, a technician can work most efficiently, yet still be able to change designs should small modifications of the restoration become necessary.

Therefore, a preliminary drawing is imperative for all prosthetic procedures and, where porcelain crowns or fixed bridges are required, the following factors must be considered:

1. The contour of the restoration must be biologically compatible with the anatomical structures in the mouth
2. A functional relationship between maxillary and mandibular teeth must exist in both static and dynamic dimensions
3. The proper thicknesses for the heterogenous materials that go into a ceramometal restoration must be defined.
4. When restoring portions of a crown or the entire crown with porcelain, the restoration must be designed to prevent shear stresses from being directed towards the junction of the porcelain with the alloy.

All necessary information sould be incorporated into the preliminary sketch. The author is accustomed to preparing what he calls a **planning wax-up** prior to the waxing procedure per se, both for single or multiple cast restoration.

Thus he incorporates all the pertinent information required above.

In this connection, it is imperative that the plan for the wax-up be based on information supplied by the dentist in the form of diagnostic models and specific instructions.

Waxing up a restoration based on a diagnostic model supplied by a dentist is known as **diagnostic wax-up,** distinguishing it from the **planning wax-up** which is used for laboratory procedures.

The following discussion centers on the various preliminary tasks which are necessary for the fabrication of wax patterns in ceramometal restorations.

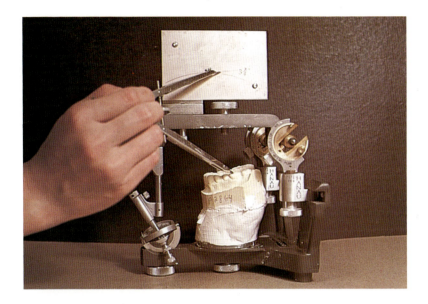

A diagnostic model prepared by a dentist (in collaboration with Dr. S. Wagman in 1964).

After studying the diagnostic model, the desired occlusal surface is registered on a plaster model, using a Broadlic Occlusal Plane Analyzer (Model 142-1, Hanau). The occlusal surface of the plaster model is cut down in accordance with the registered occlusal surface and the mandibular movement.

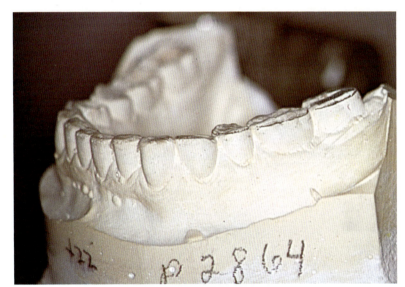

In some cases, an impression of the occlusal surfaces is made with wax. If needed, a core is reproduced from the buccolingual surface with baseplate wax. The molar retainer is fabricated using this core as a guide.

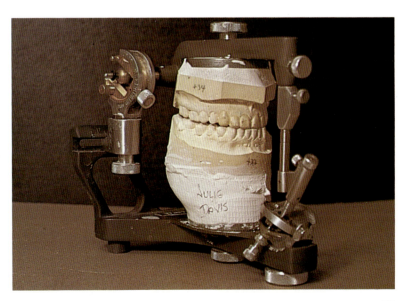

Similarly, for the anterior teeth, the crown is modified on a diagnostic model and, when necessary, wax is added with consideration of the angle of disclusion in order to increase the anterior guidance angle.

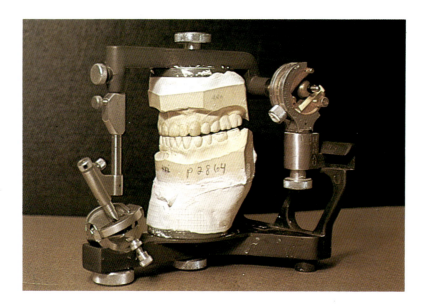

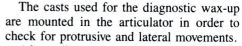

The casts used for the diagnostic wax-up are mounted in the articulator in order to check for protrusive and lateral movements.

After adjustments are completed on the model, a core is made and impressions of the anterior teeth are made. The core is used to prepare the wax-ups for the anterior teeth. The impressions taken of the anterior teeth and the molars will later be used in the fabrication of the temporary and planning crowns.

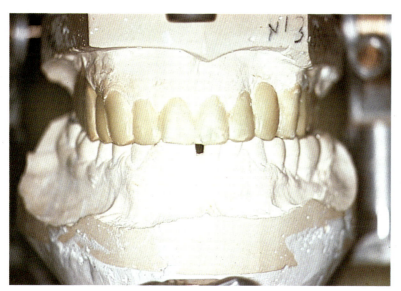

A finished diagnostic wax-up of a different case: a "planning wax up" used in a dental laboratory should be based on the diagnosis, treatment planning, and other pertinent information supplied by the dentist, which should include a working model for the fabrication of temporary crowns.

3.2 OBJECTIVES OF THE SKELETAL TECHNIQUE

As has already been stated, carefully planned preparations, with emphasis on form and function, are essential for successful restoration.

From observations of the natural teeth, we know that they are composed of three fundamental planes. Those provide us with necessary information about anatomical landmarks and the positioning of the margins of the crowns. Accordingly, our task is facilitated by having standard landmarks established.

The skeletal technique entails a method in which landmark points (cusp tips, fossa dots) are set up during the waxing process. They are joined together with wax ridges to form frames for the crown skeleton. Finally, the empty areas are filled in with wax in order to create the functionally and anatomically correct crown contour. This concept may be compared to modern building techniques. During the construction of a building, requirements of form and function are carefully studied and incorporated in the blueprints. Then the construction process, the blueprints are strictly adhered to. The blueprints set up standard points which join certain spaces together and the outer walls serve as limitations.

This series of modern buildings in Tokyo illustrate the concept of skeletal technique. In the wax-up of the incisor, the standard landmark points, line, and ridges represent the anatomical ridges of the tooth: these landmarks are called skeletal standard ridges. After these standard points and lines are set up, wax is used to fill the empty spaces between the skeletal components in order to create the three basic planes that compose the crown form.

A
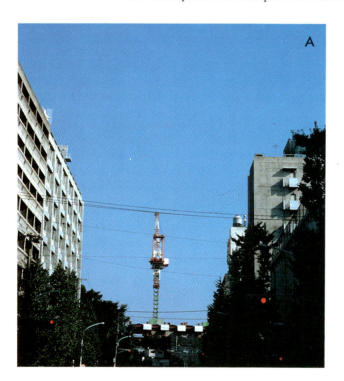

B
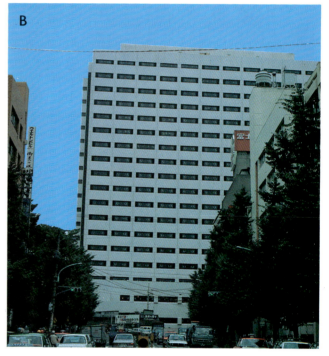

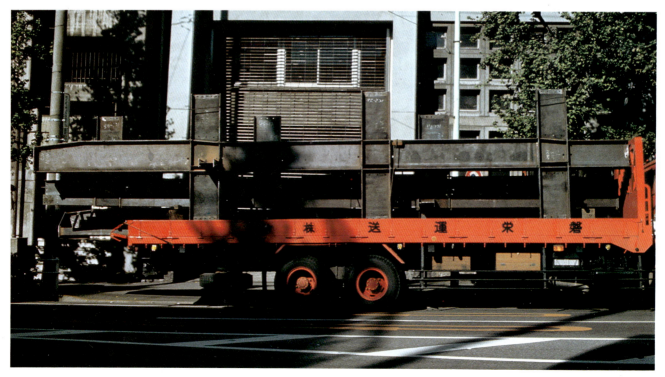

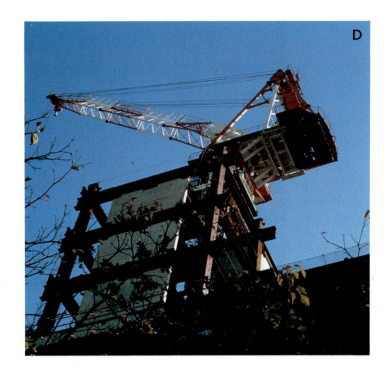

D

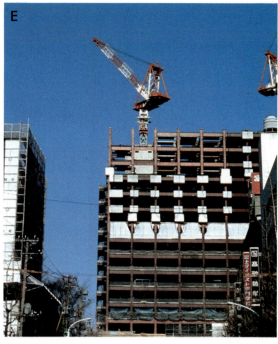

E

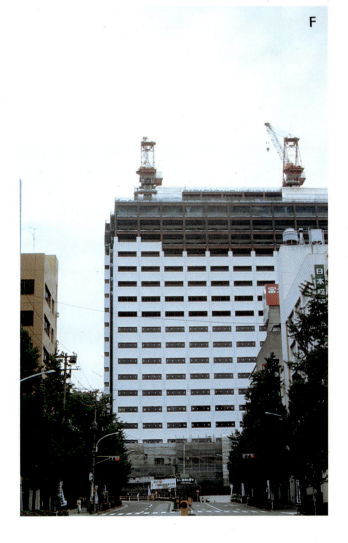

F

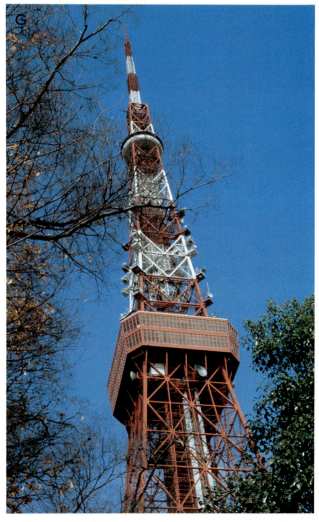

G

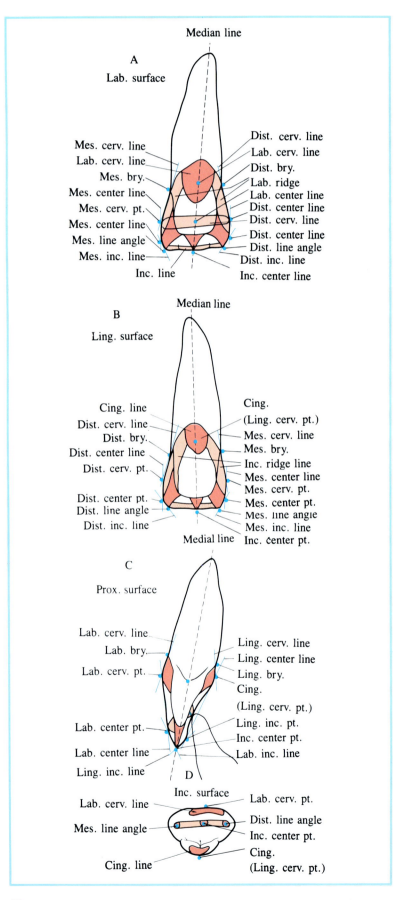

Median line

A
Lab. surface

Mes. cerv. line
Lab. cerv. line
Mes. bry.
Mes. center line
Mes. cerv. pt.
Mes. center line
Mes. line angle
Mes. inc. line
Inc. line

Dist. cerv. line
Lab. cerv. line
Dist. bry.
Lab. ridge
Lab. center line
Dist. center line
Dist. cerv. line
Dist. center line
Dist. line angle
Dist. inc. line
Inc. center line

Median line

B
Ling. surface

Cing. line
Dist. cerv. line
Dist. bry.
Dist. center line
Dist. cerv. pt.
Dist. center pt.
Dist. line angle
Dist. inc. line

Cing.
(Ling. cerv. pt.)
Mes. cerv. line
Mes. bry.
Inc. ridge line
Mes. center line
Mes. cerv. pt.
Mes. center pt.
Mes. line angle
Mes. inc. line
Inc. center pt.

Medial line

C
Prox. surface

Lab. cerv. line
Lab. bry.
Lab. cerv. pt.
Lab. center pt.
Lab. center line
Ling. inc. line

Ling. cerv. line
Ling. center line
Ling. bry.
Cing.
(Ling. cerv. pt.)
Ling. inc. pt.
Inc. center pt.
Lab. inc. line

D
Inc. surface

Lab. cerv. line
Mes. line angle
Cing. line

Lab. cerv. pt.
Dist. line angle
Inc. center pt.
Cing.
(Ling. cerv. pt.)

Boundary = bry.
Cervical = cerv.
Cingulum = cing.
Distal = dist.
Incisal = inc.
Labial = lab.
Lingual = ling.
Mesial = mes.
Point = pt.
Proximal = prox.

Boundary = bry.

Buccal = buc.

Cervical. = cerv.

Distal = dist.

Lingual = ling.

Marginal = marg.

Mesial = mes.

Occlusal = occ.

Point = pt.

Proximal = prox.

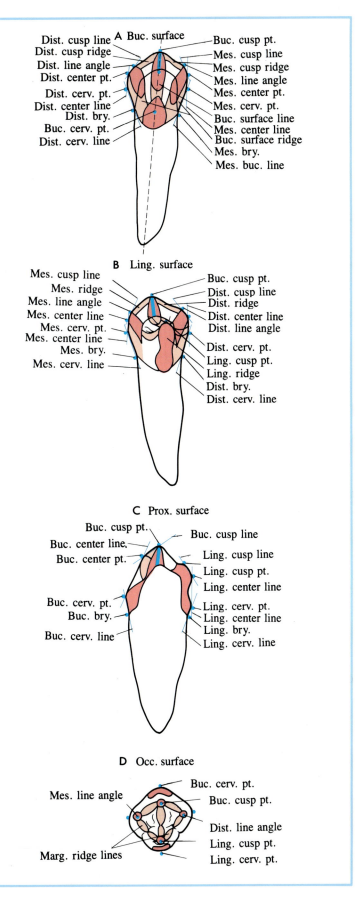

A Buc. surface

Dist. cusp line
Dist. cusp ridge
Dist. line angle
Dist. center pt.
Dist. cerv. pt.
Dist. center line
Dist. bry.
Buc. cerv. pt.
Dist. cerv. line

Buc. cusp pt.
Mes. cusp line
Mes. cusp ridge
Mes. line angle
Mes. center pt.
Mes. cerv. pt.
Buc. surface line
Mes. center line
Buc. surface ridge
Mes. bry.
Mes. buc. line

B Ling. surface

Mes. cusp line
Mes. ridge
Mes. line angle
Mes. center line
Mes. cerv. pt.
Mes. center line
Mes. bry.
Mes. cerv. line

Buc. cusp pt.
Dist. cusp line
Dist. ridge
Dist. center line
Dist. line angle
Dist. cerv. pt.
Ling. cusp pt.
Ling. ridge
Dist. bry.
Dist. cerv. line

C Prox. surface

Buc. cusp pt.
Buc. center line.
Buc. center pt.

Buc. cerv. pt.
Buc. bry.
Buc. cerv. line

Buc. cusp line
Ling. cusp line
Ling. cusp pt.
Ling. center line
Ling. cerv. pt.
Ling. center line
Ling. bry.
Ling. cerv. line

D Occ. surface

Mes. line angle

Buc. cerv. pt.
Buc. cusp pt.
Dist. line angle
Ling. cusp pt.
Ling. cerv. pt.

Marg. ridge lines

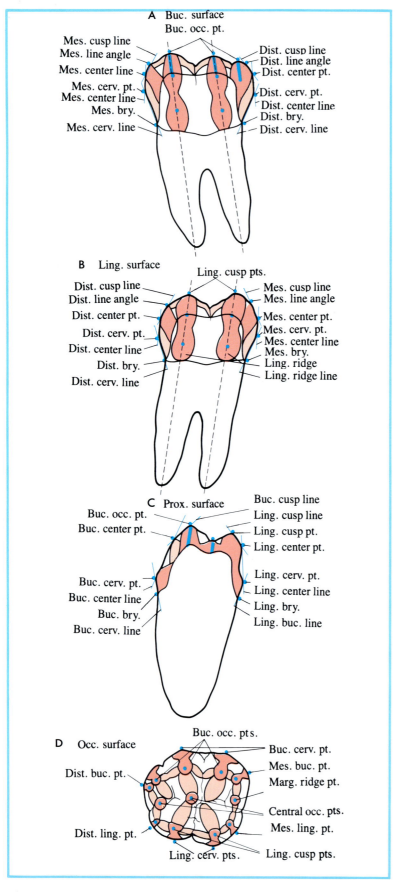

A Buc. surface
Buc. occ. pt.

Mes. cusp line
Mes. line angle
Mes. center line
Mes. cerv. pt.
Mes. center line
Mes. bry.
Mes. cerv. line

Dist. cusp line
Dist. line angle
Dist. center pt.
Dist. cerv. pt.
Dist. center line
Dist. bry.
Dist. cerv. line

B Ling. surface
Ling. cusp pts.

Dist. cusp line
Dist. line angle
Dist. center pt.
Dist. cerv. pt.
Dist. center line
Dist. bry.
Dist. cerv. line

Mes. cusp line
Mes. line angle
Mes. center pt.
Mes. cerv. pt.
Mes. center line
Mes. bry.
Ling. ridge
Ling. ridge line

C Prox. surface
Buc. occ. pt.
Buc. center pt.

Buc. cusp line
Ling. cusp line
Ling. cusp pt.
Ling. center pt.

Buc. cerv. pt.
Buc. center line
Buc. bry.
Buc. cerv. line

Ling. cerv. pt.
Ling. center line
Ling. bry.
Ling. buc. line

D Occ. surface
Buc. occ. pts.

Dist. buc. pt.

Buc. cerv. pt.
Mes. buc. pt.
Marg. ridge pt.

Central occ. pts.
Mes. ling. pt.

Dist. ling. pt.

Ling. cerv. pts.
Ling. cusp pts.

Boundary = bry.
Buccal = buc.
Cervical = cerv.
Distal = dist.
Lingual = ling.
Marginal = marg.
Mesial = mes.
Occlusal = occ.
Point = pt.
Proximal = prox.

3.3 FABRICATION OF THE WAX PATTERN: SKELETAL TECHNIQUE

The wax pattern serves as a three-dimensional blueprint for the restoration. The skeletal technique is used with the wax pattern and links together standard landmark points and lines with the basic planes, thus providing the wax skeleton. The final anatomical crown contour is obtained by filling in the missing components of the wax skeleton.

The following photographs illustrate fabrication of wax patterns for the maxillary and mandibular anterior teeth and also for the mandibular molars. Concerning the molars, the function and form of the cusp tips are most important; fine wax rods are employed for the three-dimensional wax-up. By using fine wax rods the cusp tips of the maxillary and mandibular copings are constructed. Thus, the spatial relationship between the wax crowns in the opposing arches is obtained. The functional guides that are fabricated with an anterior silicone core, the maxillary and mandibular resin canines, and the buildup of the wax crowns are necessary preliminary procedures leading to a large scale full-mouth ceramometal restoration.

3.3.1. FABRICATION OF THE WAX COPING

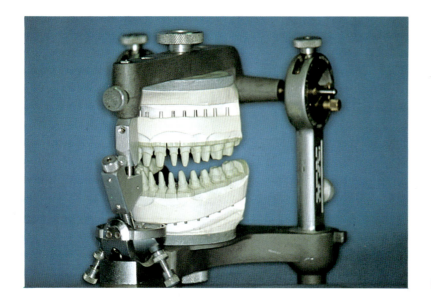

Working casts mounted on the articulator (Hanau 145-2 model).

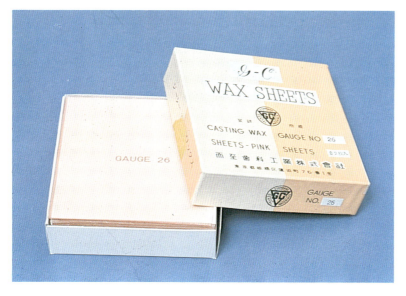

Sheet wax No. 26 (0.5mm thickness) is used for the coping.

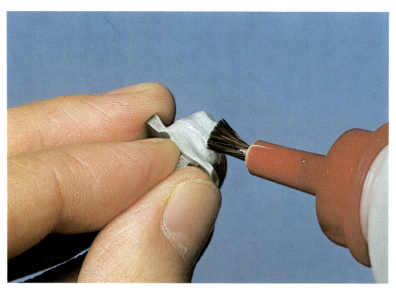

A wax separating medium is applied to the surface of the die. A separating medium which allows a uniform and thin coat should be selected.

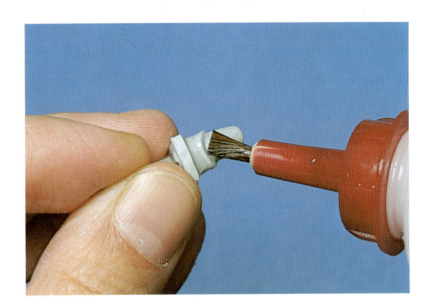

An airgun is used for the application of wax separator. Thus it is possible to obtain a uniform and thin distribution of the material on the surface.

Here the wax separating medium is applied with a brush on all tooth surfaces.

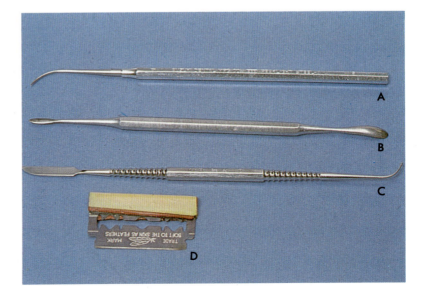

A set of instruments used for fabrication of the coping (Ishifuku Co. Ltd.).

A: Explorer
B: M.K. instrument No. 1
C: M.K. instrument No. 2
D: A double-edged razor blade

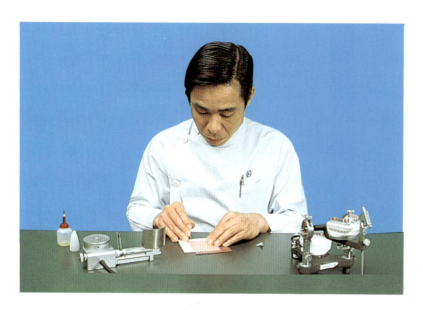

A piece of wax is cut (note basic working position #1). Note also the coordination of the right and left hand.

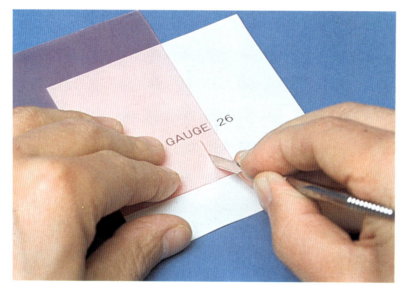

GAUGE 26

Even such a simple procedure must employ standardized digital movements.

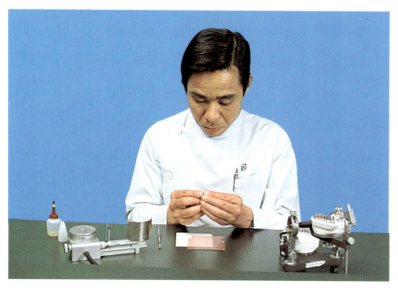

Sheet wax is adapted to the tooth surface, by using basic working position No. 2.

When adapting the piece of sheet wax to the tooth surface, the fingers are directed with the proximal areas clearly visible throughout the procedure.

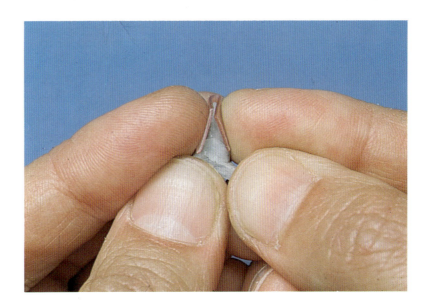

The sheet wax is adapted to the surface of the tooth.

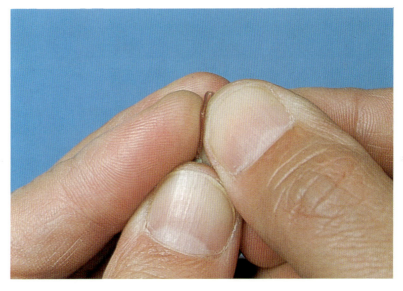

In the above finger position, the tip of the right thumb and the end of the left index finger are used to adapt the sheet wax. Thus, the wax can be adapted onto the tooth surface uniformly.

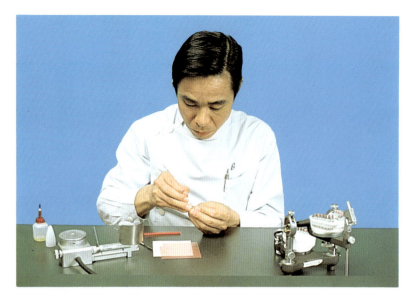

The margin of the adapted sheet wax is cut off with a carving knife in basic working position No. 3.

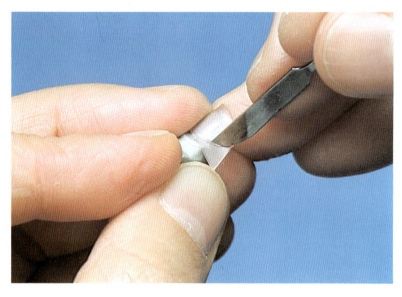

Close-up of the above.

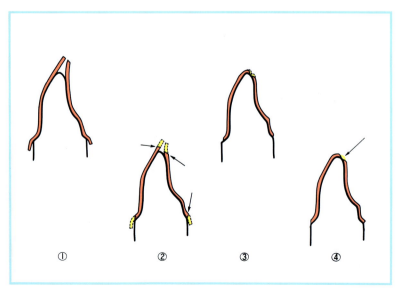

①   ②   ③   ④

Sheet wax joints are sealed in the following order:
1. Sheet wax adaptation onto the tooth surface
2. Incisal edge and margin portions are cut off
3. The incisal edge portion is bent and firmly adapted
4. The incisal edge portion is filled in with wax

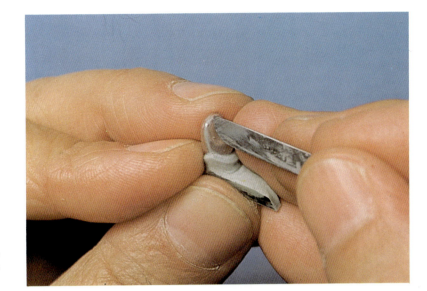

Step 3 is illustrated again. A heated carving knife is used to seal the sheet wax on the incisal edge and, at the same time, an oblique cut is made to eliminate excessive wax.

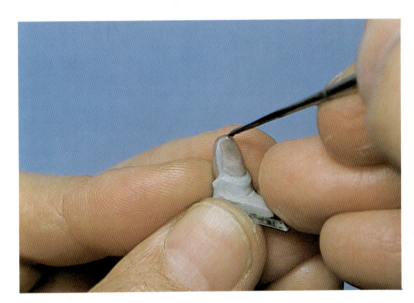

The same process is continued from the incisal edge to the proximal and cervical regions.

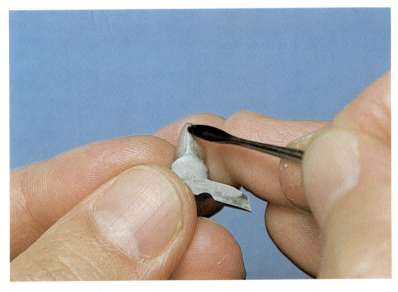

The joints are evenly filled in with additional wax.

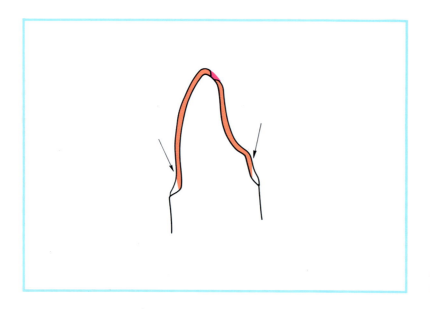

After completion of the previous step, an oblique cut is made in the marginal portion and excessive wax is then eliminated.

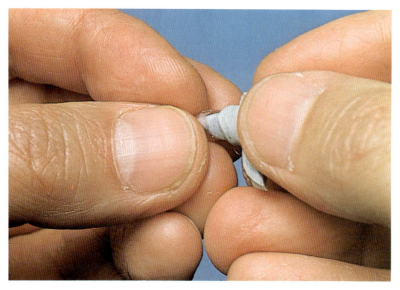

Here the wax pattern is removed from the die. Holding the die with the fingertips of the left hand, the wax pattern should be pulled out in a straight line; otherwise it will be distorted. The wax pattern is constructed on the die and should not be pulled repeatedly from the die. This will prevent distortion.

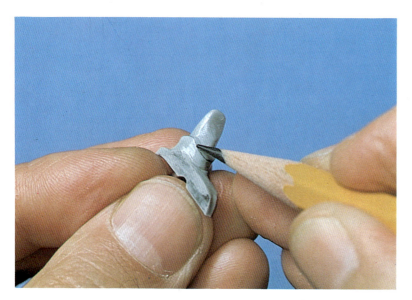

The margin line is carefully marked with a pencil, preferably under magnification. Although the margin line entry is usually made with a pencil, some other writing material, whose carbon contents will be completely eliminated during the burnout, is preferred.

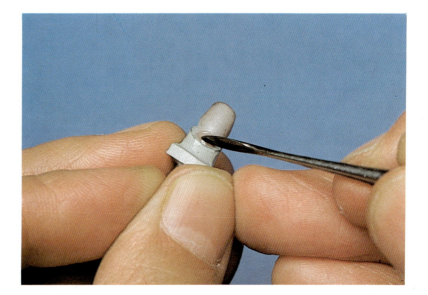

Inlay wax is added to the area between the sheet wax and the margin line.

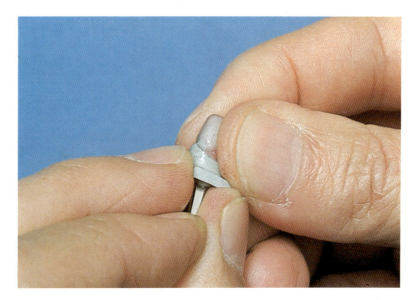

After the inlay wax has slightly cooled, it is adapted with the fingers until it sets firmly. Preparing a margin in small increments reduces the possibility of subsequent wax shrinkage to a minimum.

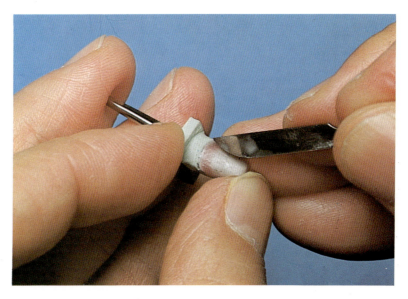

After finising the marginal area, it is carved and adjusted once more.

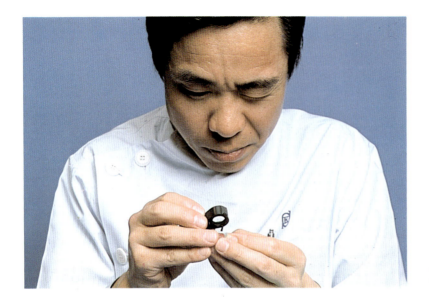

The preparation of the gingival margins is confirmed for each tooth under magnification.

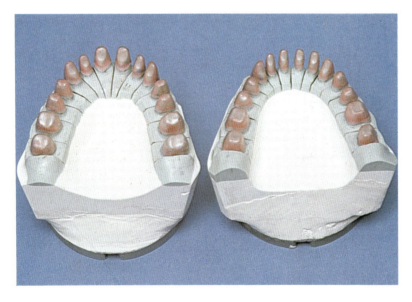

The finishing procedures for the dies of the teeth of the entire maxillary and mandibular arch are completed.

3.3.2 WAX-UP PROCEDURES FOR MAXILLARY AND MANDIBULAR ANTERIOR TEETH (SKELETAL TECHNIQUE)

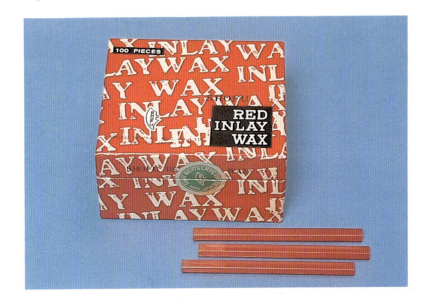

Preceding the wax-up of a crown, the selection of the correct wax is very important. A red inlay wax, marketed by Shofu Dental Co. Ltd., is shown here.

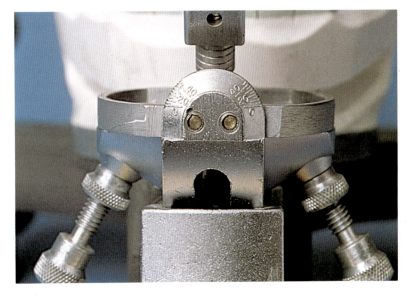

An articulator is used to record the vertical dimensions obtained from the patient's mouth. Those measurements will serve as guides during the construction of the patient's restoration. The central position of the incisal pin of the articulator is confirmed in relation to the anterior guidance table, set at 0°.

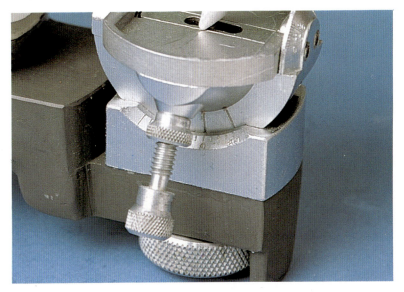

The 0° setting of the anterior guidance table is also confirmed sagittally.

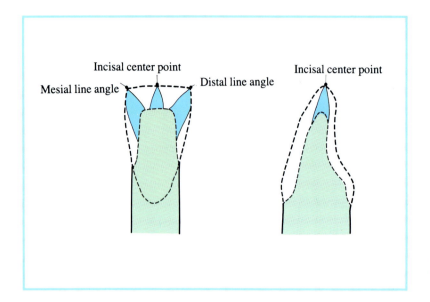

Incisal center point

Mesial line angle Distal line angle

Incisal center point

The first step of this procedure entails setting up center points for the mandibular central incisor edges and the mesial and distal line angle points.

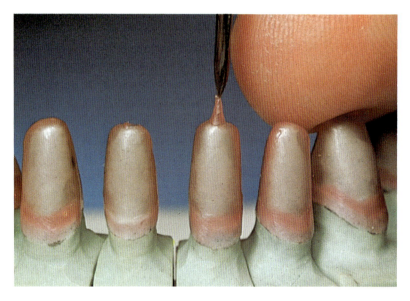

When seen sagittally, the incisal edges, the interdental papillae, and the root tips are nearly on a straight (imaginary) line. The incisal center of the die covered with sheet wax coincides in height with the line between the incisal edges.

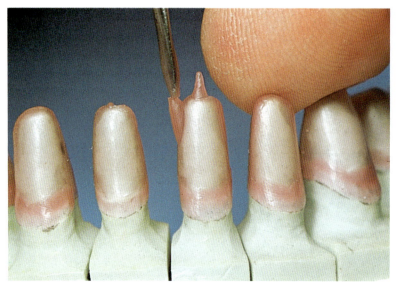

Then a standard point for the mesial and distal line angle is established by taking into account the length and width of the crown on both sides of the skeletal plane.

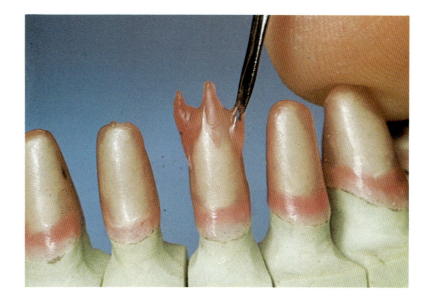

Similar to the preceding illustration, the mesial and distal line angles are set up here.

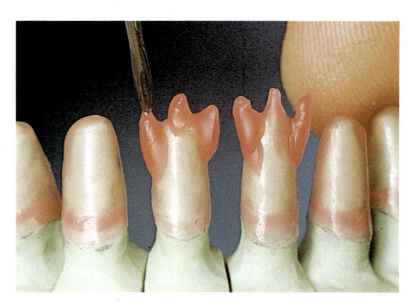

The right mandibular central incisor is treated in the same manner.

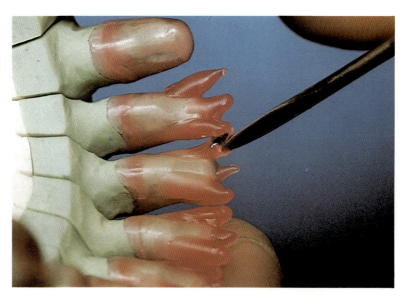

When the four mandibular incisors are finished, the alignment of the incisors is adjusted as needed.

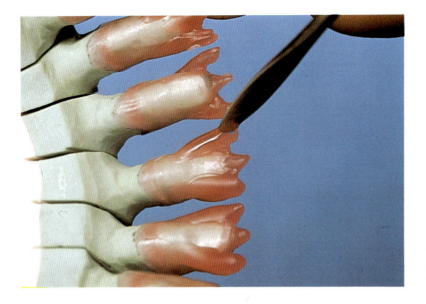

At this point, the mesial line angle of the central incisor is joined with the distal line angle of the central incisor to confirm whether the distance between the two points is adequate. A prior estimation of the correct position of the point will be helpful.

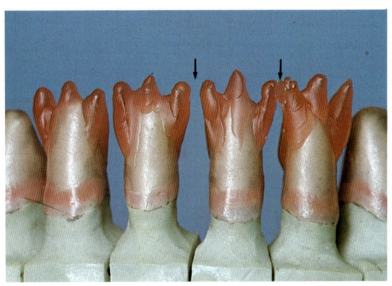

Here, the distance between the two points is adequate.

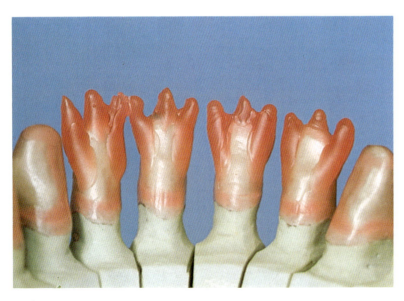

The distance is also confirmed from the lingual side. The three planes are adequate means for determining the external outline of the crown, which is completed at a later date.

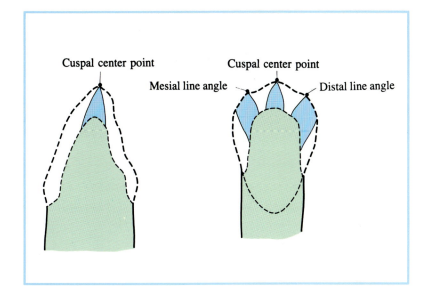

Cuspal center point   Cuspal center point

Mesial line angle   Distal line angle

The cuspal center line of the mandibular canine and its mesiodistal line angle are diagrammed here.

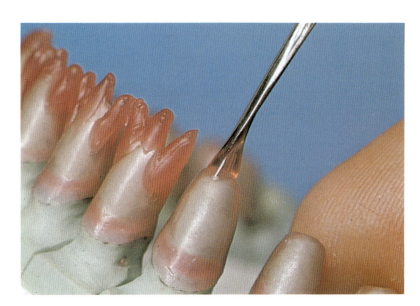

When looking at the canine, the three points are also more or less on a straight line, and therefore, a standard point is set up on the ridge center.

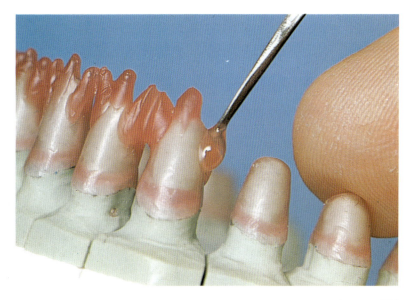

Subsequently, the mesiodistal line angle of the canine is established, considering canine contour and curvature of the dental arch.

When the mesiodistal line angles are established on all mandibular anterior teeth, the line angle points are proximally joined.

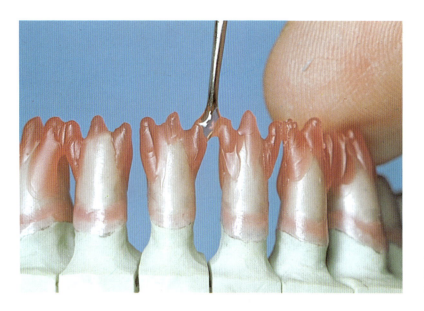

By joining the proximal line angle points, we can estimate the crown widths and proximal distances that are created in the final stage.

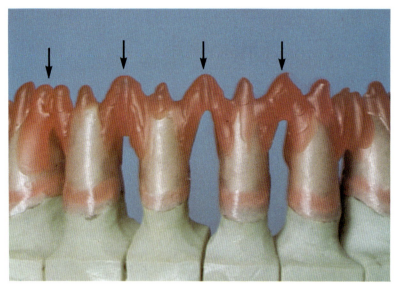

The wax-up is continued with periodic checking of the occlusal relationship between the maxillary and mandibular teeth.

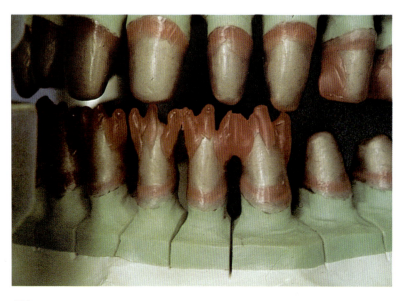

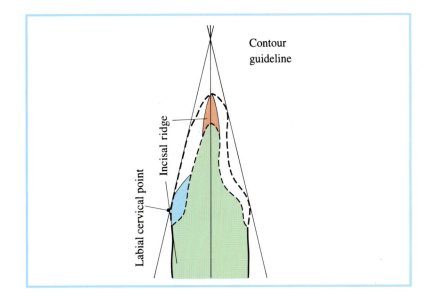

The labial cervical point is established for the mandibular anterior teeth. This point is established according to the three plane concept and the contour guideline.

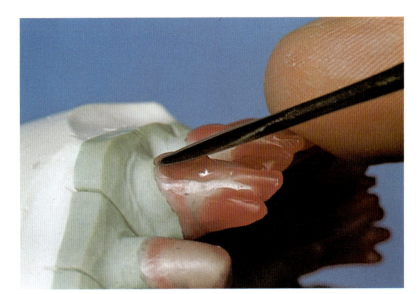

With the mandibular anterior teeth, the labial height of contour is found on a line which runs from the long axis of the tooth to the area of the greatest labio-lingual crown width. This fact is used to establish the labial cervical line and the standard point.

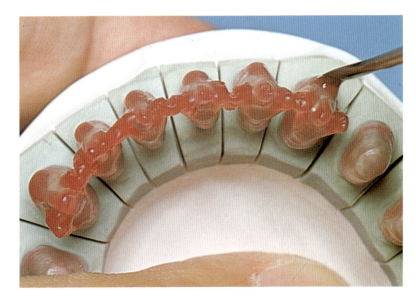

The labial cervical point is an important feature. The labial cervical ridge is built up to harmonize with gingival contour in order to guarantee harmony with the gingival tissues.

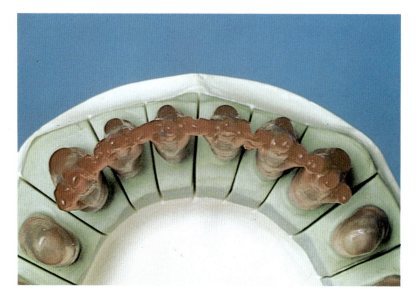

This photograph shows the mandibular anterior teeth after completion of the procedure shown above. This wax-up provides us with important information concerning the crown contour of the mandibular anterior teeth and their relation to the rest of the dental arch. Here it is important that the distal line angles of the canines are in alignment with the buccolingual center of the premolars and molars.

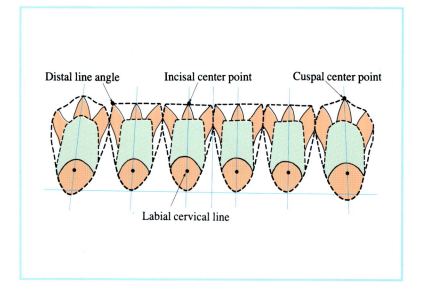

The standard points set up for the mandibular anterior teeth.

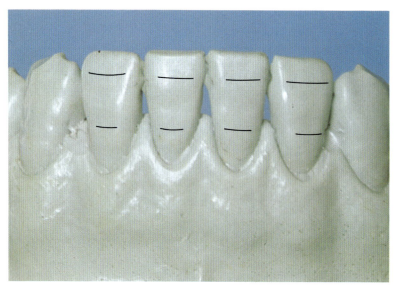

The positional relationships of the mandibular anterior teeth are now being verified on the natural dentition of the mandibular arch.

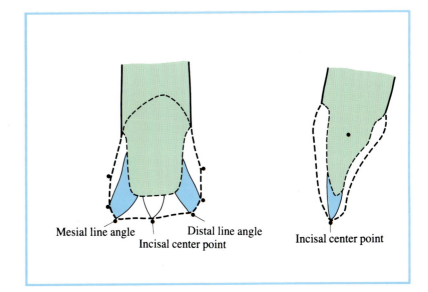

Mesial line angle   Distal line angle   Incisal center point
                   Incisal center point

In the maxillary arch, the mesiodistal line angle of the central incisor is established. The incisal edge center point is marked.

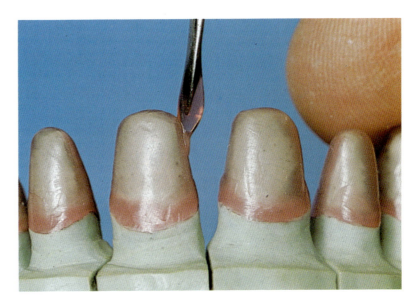

The incisal edge point and the mesiodistal line angles must be aligned on a straight line when viewed from the incisal edges.

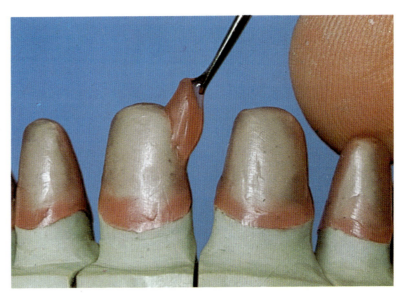

The wax-up of the mesial line angle on the maxillary left central incisor, determining the mesial line angle point.

111

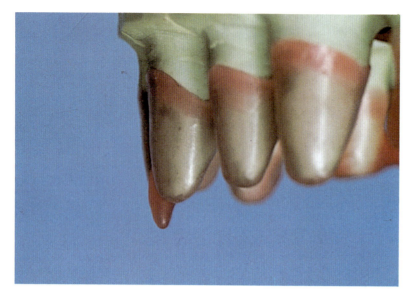

Occlusal contact between the maxillary incisal ridge line and the mandibular incisal edge is essential. Accordingly, when constructing the skeletal structure for the maxillary incisal edge, the mesiodistal point should be established so that the mutual relationship between the maxillary and mandibular arches can be determined visually.

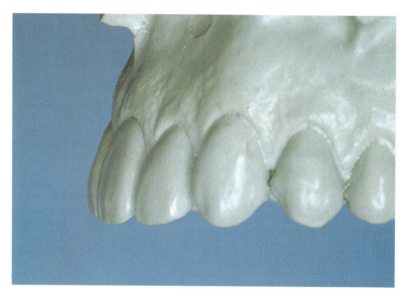

Either the mesiodistal line angle point or an incisal center point is enough to establish the basis of the three-plane construction.

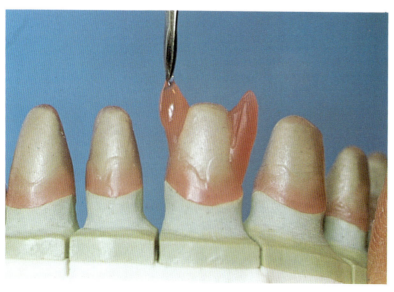

The distal line angles are established for the remaining maxillary incisors.

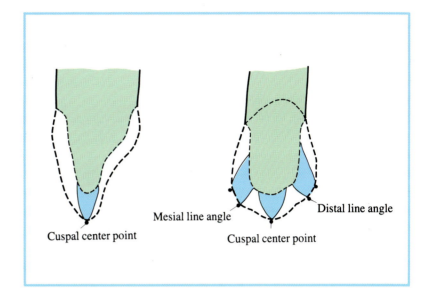

Cuspal center point

Mesial line angle   Distal line angle

Cuspal center point

After the four line angles for the maxillary incisors are established, the maxillary cuspal center point and the mesiodistal line angle point are set up for the canine.

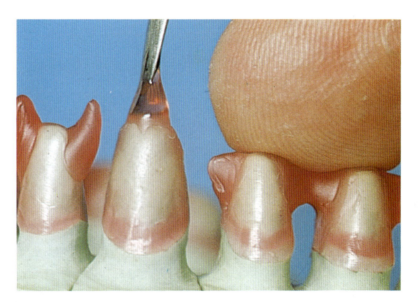

By constructing the cusp tip, the center point is established on the maxillary canine. Since the cusp center is crucial anatomically, this point must be established first.

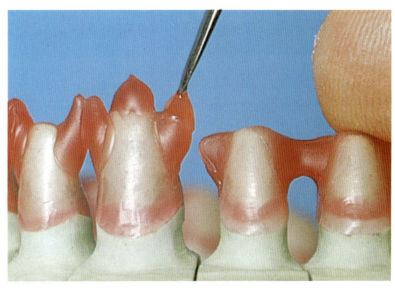

The mesiodistal line angles are established on the maxillary canine. The triangular contour of the canine cusp tip is determined from the position of the mesiodistal center point and its height.

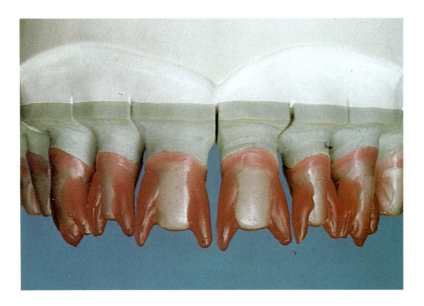

A labial view of the maxillary anterior teeth. As the alignment of the anterior teeth is determined by a line which joins the respective mesiodistal line angles with the cuspal center line, the respective mesiodistal line angles are adjusted mesially and distally, labio-lingually.

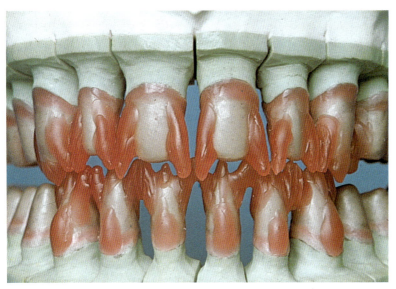

The above procedure is verified by occluding the maxillary and mandibular anterior teeth in the articulator. Here we are observing the functional lengths of the crowns and the esthetic contour of the dental arches in centric relation occlusion. All information relating to the anterior guidance of this patient can hereby be incorporated and checked.

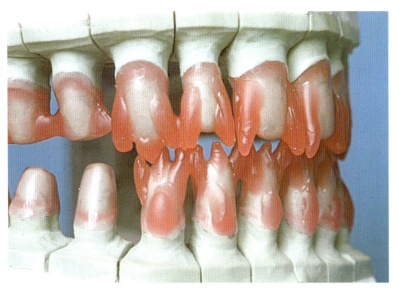

A view of the right side. As the center line of the incisal edge is absent at this stage, the relationship between the maxillary and mandibular arches can be easily observed.

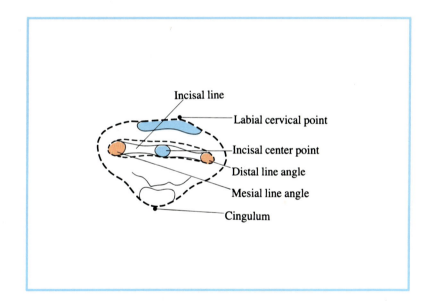

The gingival line of healthy gingival tissue along the maxillary incisors and canines is not semi-lunar in form, but resembles a zonal triangle with its tip placed distally. Therefore, the labial cervical point should be positioned there (Dr. R.S. Stein).

Incisal line

Labial cervical point

Incisal center point

Distal line angle

Mesial line angle

Cingulum

The labial height of contour, which is so important to gingival health, coincides with a vertical line from the tip of this zonal triangle.

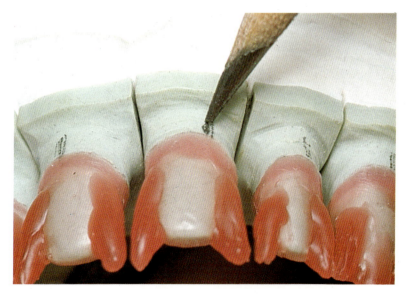

The respective positions of the zonal triangles are registered on a working model.

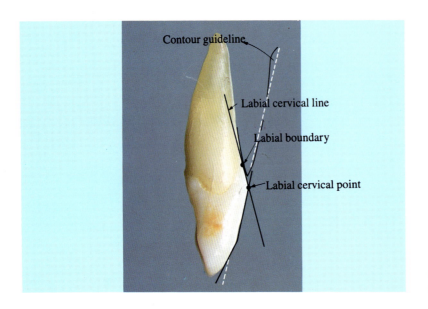

Contour guideline

Labial cervical line

Labial boundary

Labial cervical point

The labial cervical point is established by referring to the three basic planes and the crown contour.

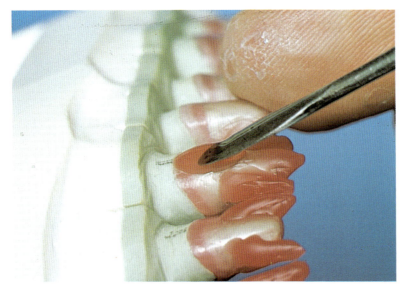

The labial height of contour is built up, and will serve as a guide for the labial cervical point and the labial cervical line. Careful attention is necessary here, because the labial cervical point positioned on the height of contour is an important factor for the functional transition between crown and root surfaces and gingival tissues.

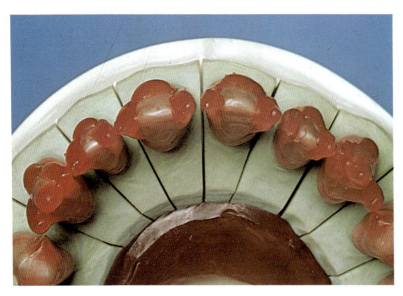

An incisal view of the waxed maxillary anteriors, with the mesiodistal line angle point and labial cervical point showing. Establishing the major skeleton helps us to achieve an outline form for the anterior teeth and for part of the remaining dental arch.

The incisal center point of the maxillary incisors is subsequently set up to the mesiodistal line angle point established previously. Thus it is possible to know the position of the center of the labial crown surface in advance, which makes it easy to establish the height of contour.

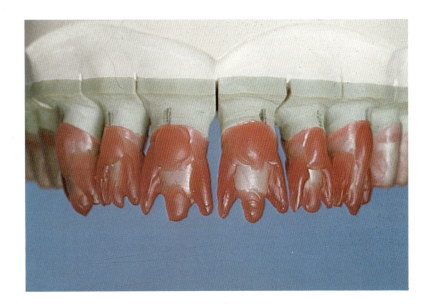

A later stage of our wax-up, in which the mesiodistal line angle point and the incisal center point are joined. The mesiodistal line angle point, the cuspal center point, the labial cervical point and the incisal center point are thus established for the maxillary anterior teeth.

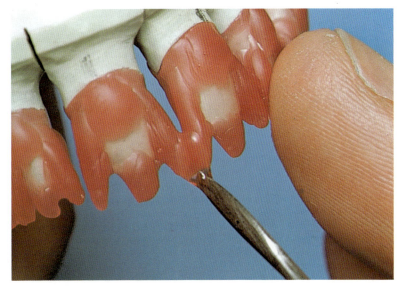

The line angle points of the maxillary anterior teeth are again joined with wax; this helps the technician to anticipate the ultimate width of the dental arch and the respective positions of these teeth.

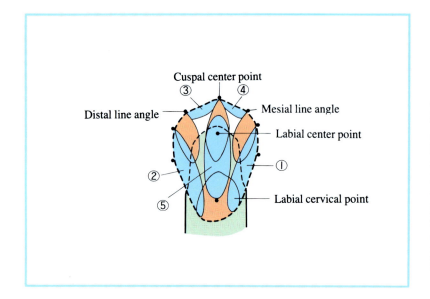

Cuspal center point

③ ④

Distal line angle — Mesial line angle

— Labial center point

② ①

⑤ — Labial cervical point

As the next step, respective landmark points are joined with wax. Since the mandibular premolars play a central role in the entire arch form, the procedure is shown here. First, the labial cervical and the mesiodistal line angle points are linked to the labial cusp ridge, as in ① and ②. The mesiodistal line angle point and the cuspal center point are connected through the mesial and distal cusp ridge, as in ③ and ④. The labial cervical ridge and the cuspal center ridge are joined together through the labial center ridge, as in ⑤.

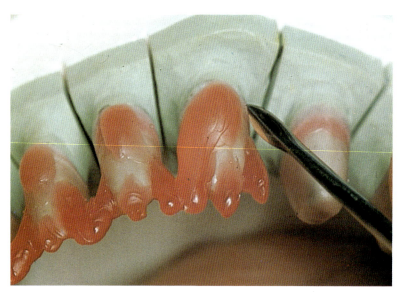

After the labial cervical point and the mesial line angle point of the mandibular canines are linked together, a distal line angle is waxed up.

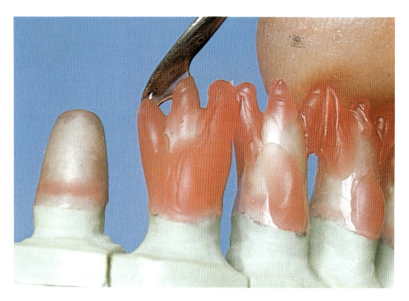

Subsequently, the distal line angle point and the cuspal center point are joined together with the cuspal ridge.

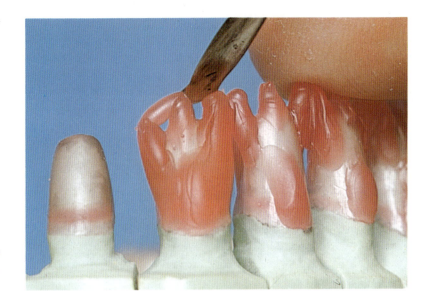

The mesial line angle and the cuspal center point are joined with wax. This procedure is completed in one continuous operation.

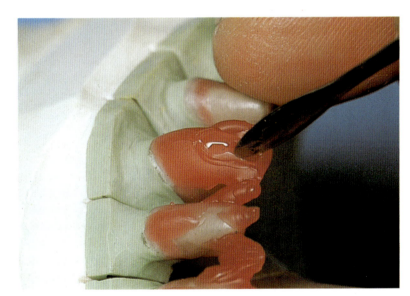

After the labial cervical point and incisal center point are joined, the lateral outline form of the mandibular canine is obtained. The well developed central cusp ridge must be emphasized on this tooth. By filling in the respective landmark ridges with wax, the anatomical form is roughly outlined.

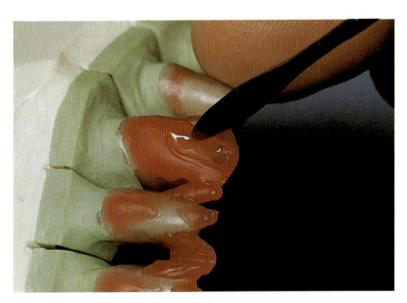

For convenience's sake, the procedure is divided into two stages: during the first, the distal side and during the second, the mesial side of the canine are waxed up.

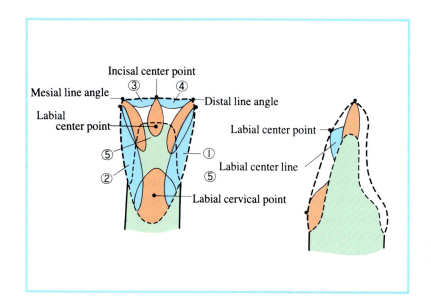

As shown previously on the canine, the respective landmarks of the mandibular incisors are joined with wax. The labial cervical point and the mesial and distal line angle points are connected through the labial cusp ridge, as in ① and ②. Now the mesial and distal line angles and the cuspal center point are linked, as in ③ and ④, and finally the labial center point is established by building up the labial central ridge, as in ⑤.

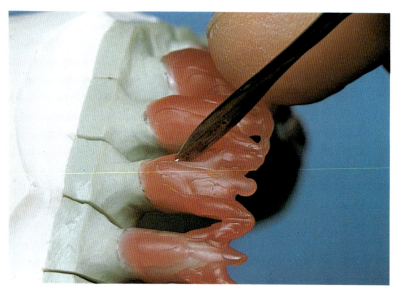

A view of the mandibular lateral right incisor, with steps one to four completed.

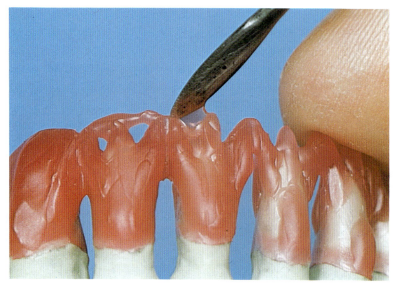

The distal line angle and the cuspal center point on the mandibular right central incisor are linked through the incisal ridge.

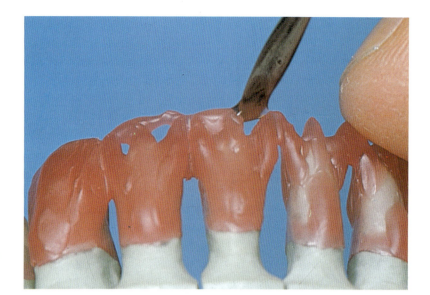

The incisal center point and the mesial line angle are joined together. After the respective landmark points of the incisors have been waxed and joined, the same procedure is performed on the canines of the opposite side.

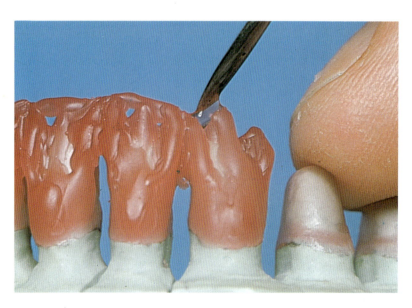

Here, the mesial line angle and the cuspal center point are linked through the incisal ridge.

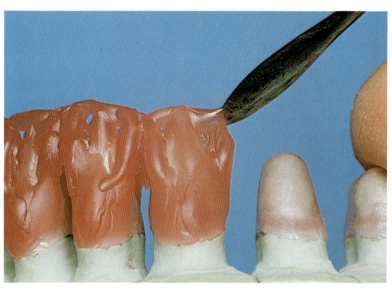

The distal line angle and the cuspal center point are joined through the incisal ridge.

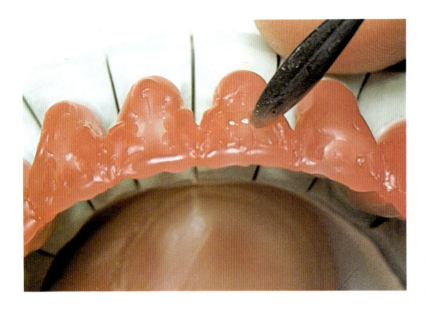

The labial center ridge is built up to obtain the labial center point for the mandibular central incisors. The point is set as a contour guideline.

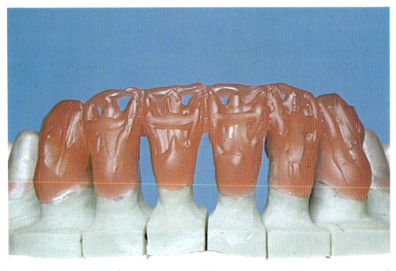

A labial view of the mandibular incisors. Since the functional and esthetic requirements have been fully incorporated in the initial planning, the crown contour can be obtained by simply filling in the skeletons without any further wax carving.

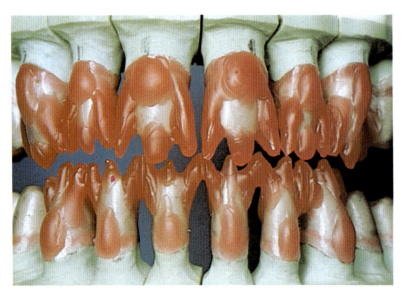

A labial view of the mandibular and maxillary anterior teeth in protrustion.

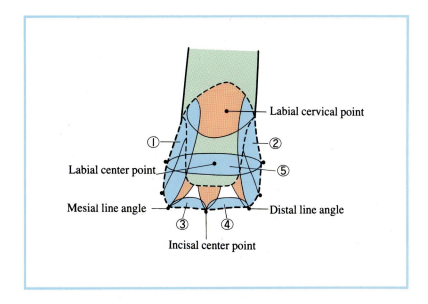

The respective landmark points of the maxillary incisors are linked together. The labial cervical point and the mesial and distal line angles are joined through the labial ridge, as in ① and ②. The mesial and distal line angles and the incisal center point are joined incisally as in ③ and ④. Finally, the labial center point is established by building up the labial center point ⑤. Here, esthetic considerations must receive special attention.

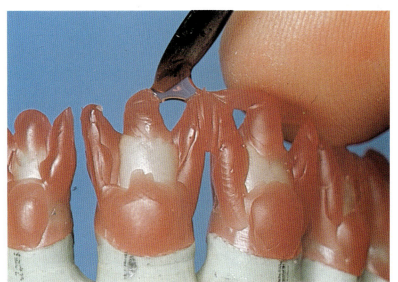

The mesial line angle and the incisal center point are joined through the incisal ridge to help estimate the future contour of the labial ridge (① — ④).

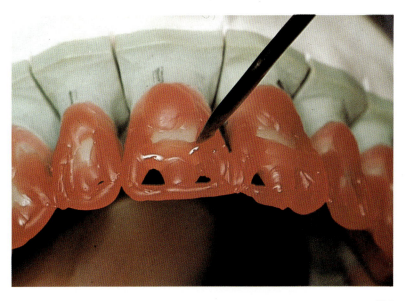

Subsequently, the labial center point is established by building up the labial central ridge. In this procedure, the contour is carried out tentatively, taking into consideration the three basic planes that will form the entire structure.

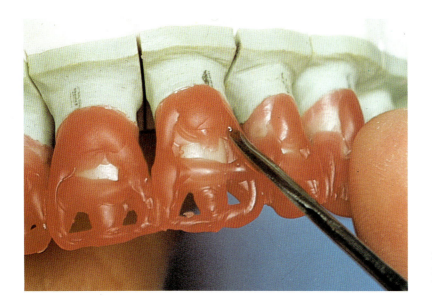

After the labial center point is set up, the mesial and distal ridge contours are adjusted, in keeping with the facial features characteristic of the patient.

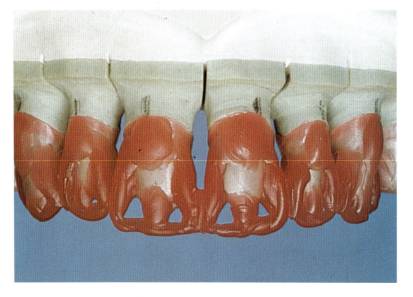

The labiolingual, upward, and downward positions of the labial center ridges have much bearing on the esthetic appearance of the final restoration. A labial view of the maxillary anteriors after completion of the procedure illustrated above.

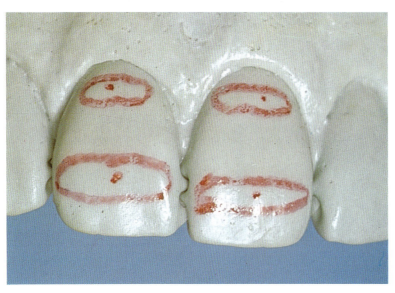

The labial cervical points and the labial center points of the maxillary central incisors are compared here.

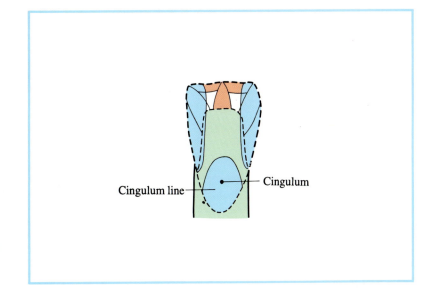

Cingulum line — • — Cingulum

On the lingual surface of the mandibular incisor, the cingulum is established and the incisal edge line is formed. The cingulum is set up nearly in the center of the mesio-distal width and a functional contact with the opposing teeth is attempted.

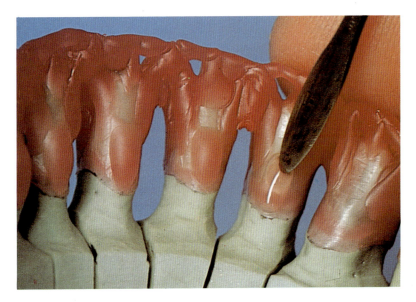

The margingal ridge lines are established parallel to each other and are not as pronounced as on the maxillary incisors.

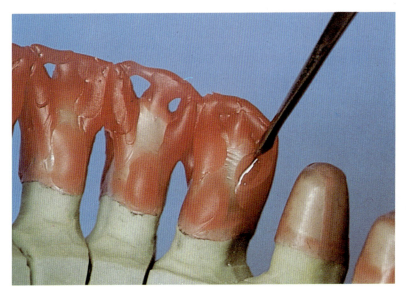

The marginal ridge lines are established for the mandibular canines. Compared with the maxillary canines, these are less developed.

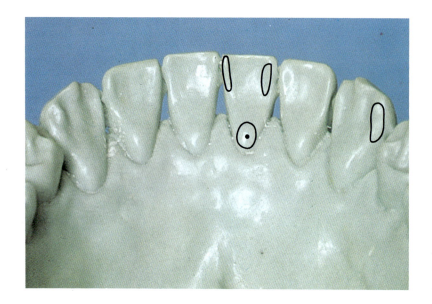

A lingual view of the mandibular anterior teeth on a cast of the natural dentition. The morphological characteristics of the cingulum and marginal ridges are well defined.

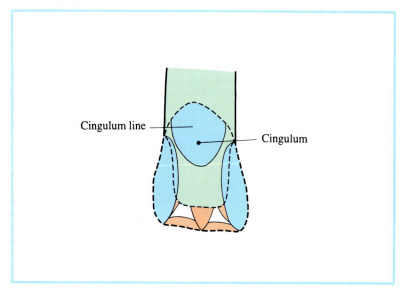

Cingulum line

Cingulum

On the lingual surface of the maxillary incisor, the form of the marginal ridge line — previously established in connection with the labial mesial and distal line angles — is touched up.

The mesial and distal ridge lines are constructed parallel to each other, longer than ½ of the tooth length and in an occlusal relationship with the mandibular teeth.

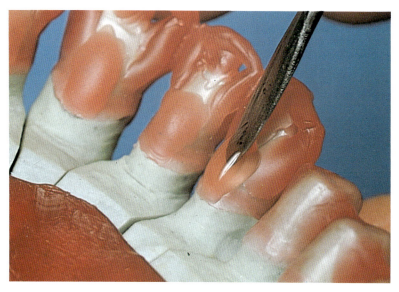

By building up the cingulum, the cingulum ridge line, which is nearly in the center of the crown as on the mandibular incisors, is created. Because the ridges are more pronounced on the maxillary incisors, the lingual contour appears to be spoon shaped.

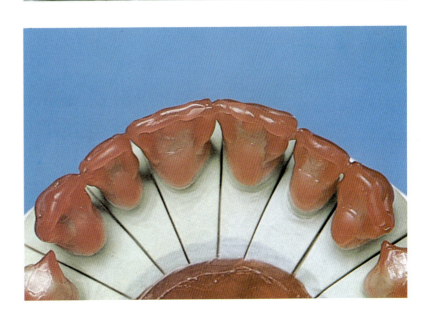

The lingual view of the maxillary anterior teeth on a cast of the natural dentition. Differences in the degree of development of the maxillary and mandibular anterior teeth and their morphological characteristics can be observed.

In accordance with the factors mentioned above, the basic morphological characteristics are now reproduced in wax.

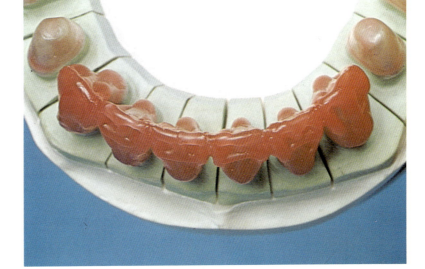

An incisal view of the mandibular anterior teeth.

The skeletal relationships, including outer labial and lingual surface contours, the respective positional relations of the teeth, occlusal contacts, the degree of maxillary overjet, and the contacts between upper and lower lips at the time of the opening of the mouth are carefully examined.

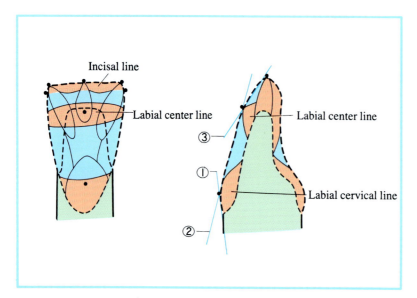

Incisal line

Labial center line

③

①

②

Labial center line

Labial cervical line

In this illustration, spatial landmark points are established by building up ridges on the maxillary and mandibular anterior teeth. This facilitates the wax-up. The procedure starts from the lateral labial side of the mandibular anterior teeth in an order of ①, ②, and ③. One was previously established when the labial cervical point was determined.

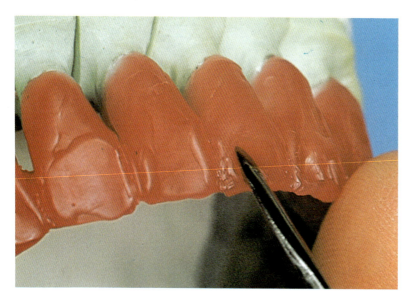

A labial view of the mandibular anterior teeth. Two planes are established by filling in the space between the labial cervical ridge and the labial center ridge, and the ridge between the incisal and the labial center ridge.

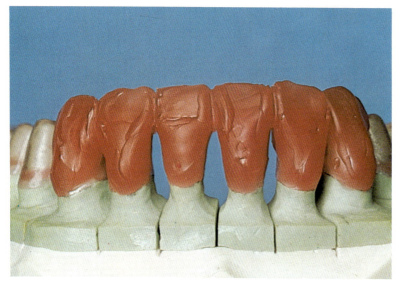

Three planes are created by filling in the respective ridge spaces of the six mandibular anterior teeth. Subsequently, a lingual plane is established in the area between the mesiodistal marginal ridge and the cingulum.

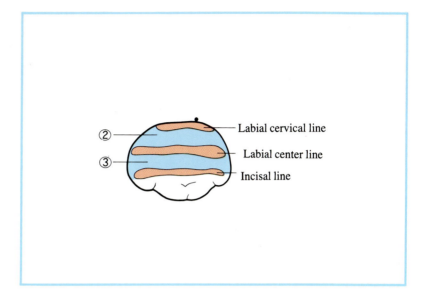

② ——— Labial cervical line

③ ——— Labial center line

Incisal line

The labial surface of the maxillary anterior teeth is composed of two planes, ② and ③. At this stage, the lingual surface is not yet prepared.

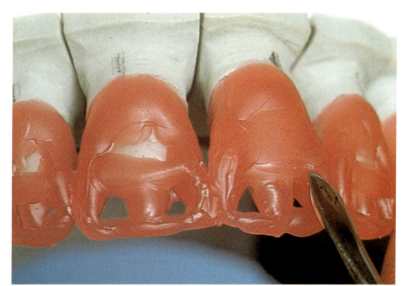

On the maxillary left central incisor, the area between the labial cervical ridge and the labial center ridge is filled in with wax. Also, the labial plane is filled in with wax.

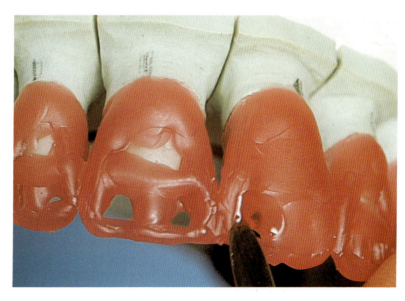

The mesial area between the incisal ridge and the labial center ridge is filled in.

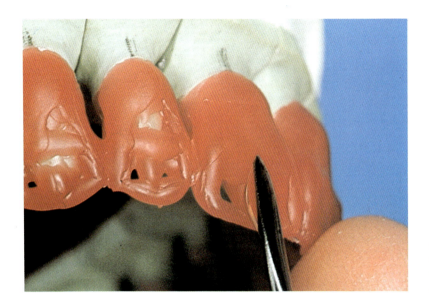

Subsequently, the labial surface of the maxillary right central incisor is filled in with wax in order to connect the labial cervical ridge and the labial center ridge. The procedure is completed at this time.

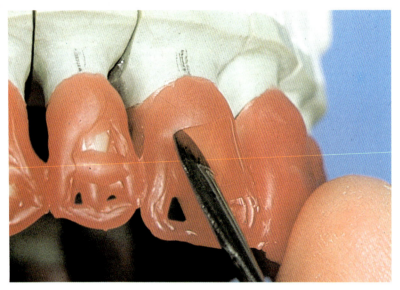

The contour of the labial surface is nearly finished.

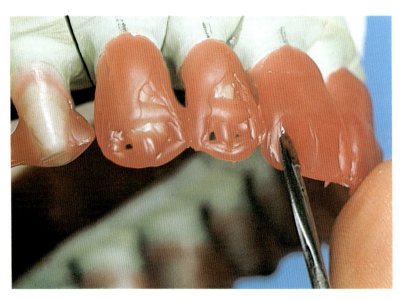

The three planes constituting the labial surface can thus be easily obtained without any further wax carving.

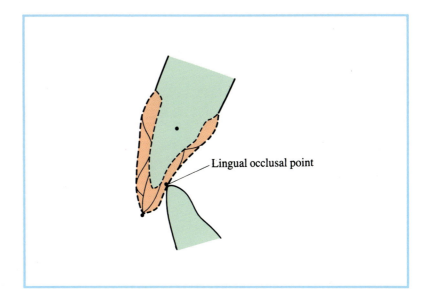

Lingual occlusal point

A lingual occlusal contact point is set up on the maxillary incisor in order to establish the correct occlusal relationship with the mandibular anterior teeth.

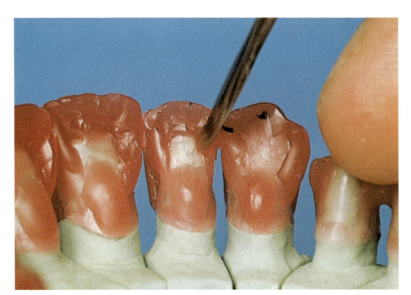

The maxillary ridge lines are adjusted for correct alignment with the mandibular anterior teeth, in centric relation/occlusion.

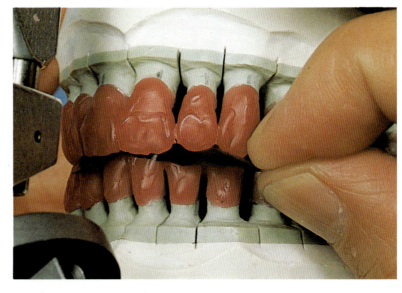

After mounting the models on the articulator, the maxillary and mandibular casts are brought into occlusal contact. Without disturbing the vertical relations previously recorded on the articulator, the contact areas between the mandibular incisal edges and the maxillary incisal ridge lines are recorded.

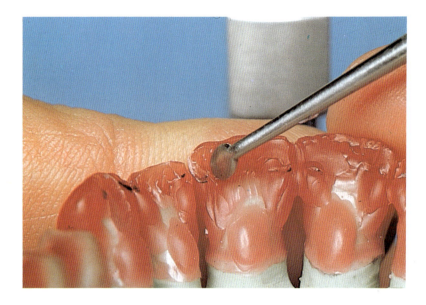

The wax portions which do not come into contact during closing of the articulator are removed at this time.

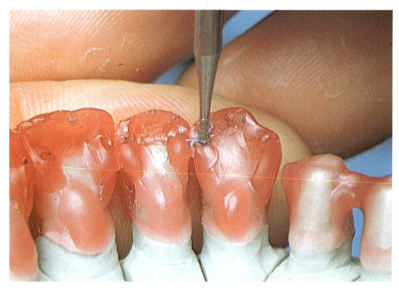

Using a 0.8-1.0mm fissure or round bur, holes are drilled into the previously indicated contact areas. The holes must not reach the tooth surfaces. The purpose of these holes is to take an accurate record of the maxillary and mandibular anterior contacts with wax rods, (0.7mm in diameter). The completion of these holes is continued with the rest of the anterior teeth.

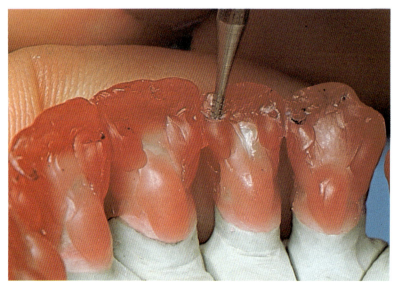

The holes are drilled on the mesial marginal ridge line for the maxillary left lateral incisor.

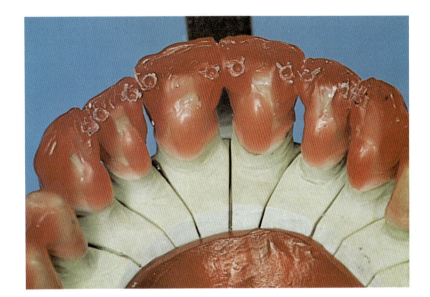

A lingual view of the waxed-up maxillary anterior teeth with all the perforations completed.

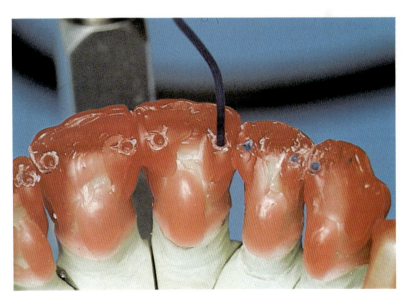

0.7mm wax rods are inserted into the respective holes.

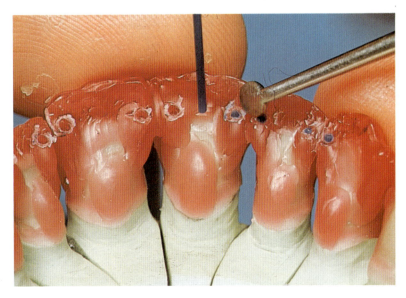

The inserted wax rods are left somewhat longer and then trimmed off. Some pressure is applied and the wax stubs are completely embedded in the holes.

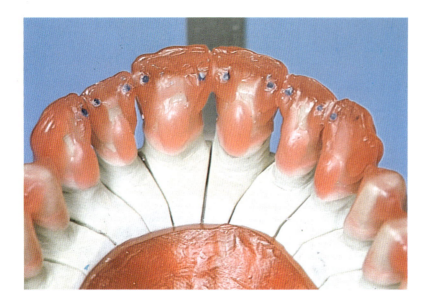

The wax rods have been inserted and thus the occlusal contacts of both the maxillary and the mandibular anteriors can be accurately recorded. These rods can also be used on the planning crowns for determination of the boundary between porcelain and metal during the wax-up. They provide us with reliable guides for occlusal relationships of the teeth during the porcelain build-up.

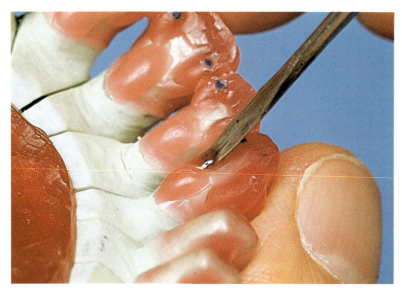

Based on the information referring to their occlusal relationships, the lingual surfaces of the maxillary incisors are filled in with wax between the marginal ridges, the cingulum, and the incisal ridges.

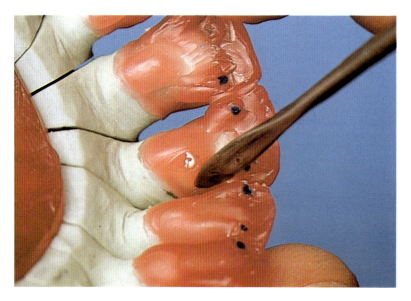

The area between the cingulum and the distal marginal ridge on the maxillary left central incisor is filled in with wax.

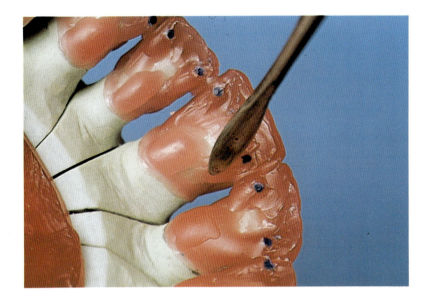

In the next step, the area between the cingulum and the distal marginal ridge line is filled in on the right central incisor.

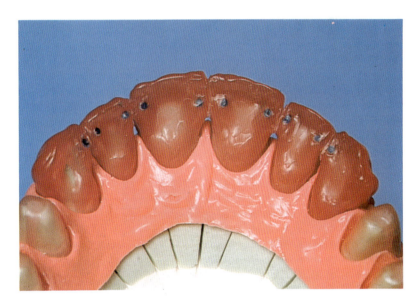

The interproximal embrasures are formed. Using the soft gingiva model as a reference, the gingival contour is finished.

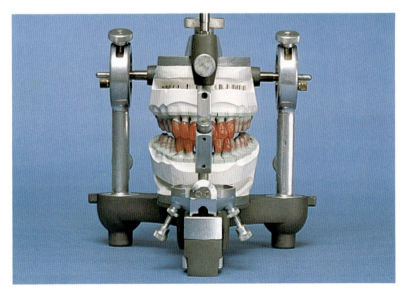

The completed crowns, based on the skeletal technique, (labial view) maxillary and mandibular anterior teeth.

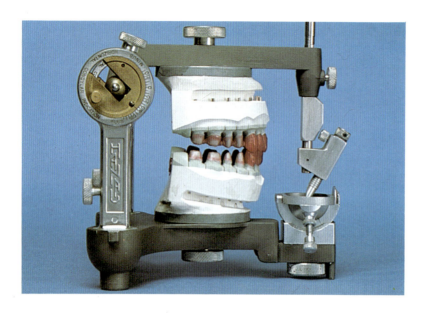

3.3.3 ANTERIOR GUIDANCE DESIGN

After the diagnostic wax-up has been completed (as illustrated previously), the work proceeds with the design of the anterior guidance. The dentist's information, based on intraoral findings in addition to information from the diagnostic casts, helps to determine the vertical relationship between maxillary and mandibular arches. This finding is transferred onto the wax crown of the casts. Since the wax is not strong enough to withstand any impact, it is necessary to protect the wax copings by using the anterior guidance of the incisal table. The articulator used here is the Hanau 145-2 type and its anterior guidance table is set at 0°.

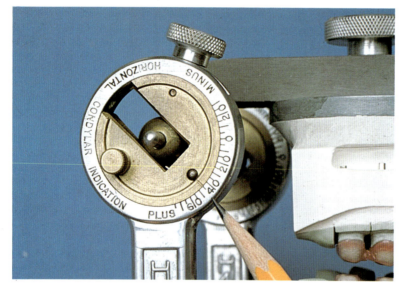

In this case, the right and left sagittal condylar paths are found to be 45°.

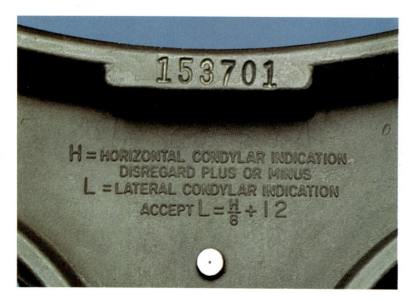

With this type of semi-adjustable articulator, the lateral condylar inclination which is clinically acceptable is computed as a mean of the value of the horizontal condylar inclination x $\frac{1}{8}$ + 12. Since the horizontal condylar inclination gives a value of 45°, the equation will be as follows:

Left condylar inclination $\frac{45}{8} + 12 = 17.6°$

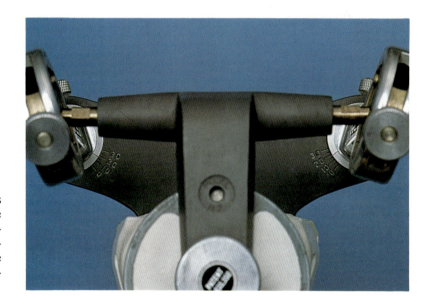

Based on the above equation, the right lateral condylar angle is adjusted to 17.6°. A similar adjustment is made on the left side. When the condylar inclinations are different on the right and left side, adjustments can be made using the formula $L = \dfrac{H}{8} + 12$ for any given case.

The right and left condylar angles are thus adjusted. When a lateral movement is made with this semi-adjustable articulator, the condylar head moves on the balancing side, forming an angle. The proper manipulation of the articulator itself is a prerequisite for all procedures discussed in this volume.

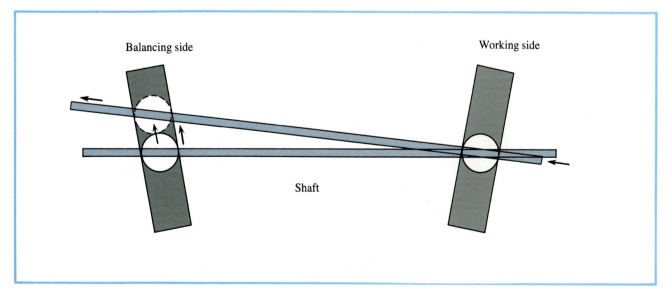

Balancing side

Working side

Shaft

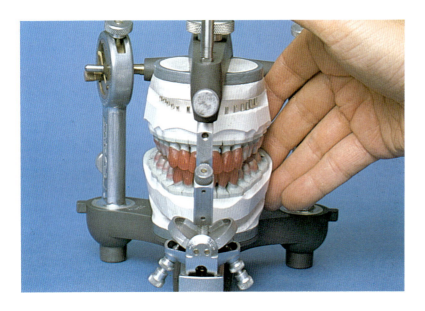

Proper finger manipulation is shown for right lateral movement of the mandible. The anterior angle (derived from the dentists's clinical information) is set for the incisal table, and then the right middle, ring, and little finger are placed firmly on the backside of the mandibular cast and the articulator.

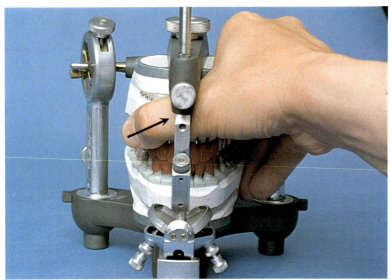

The labial side of the maxillary cast is held with the apex of the right thumb. The thumb's tip is also used to protect the right canine. The arrow indicates the direction of movement.

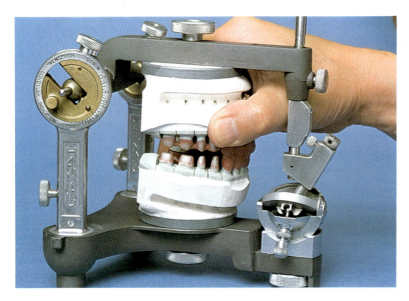

A lateral view of the same procedure. Note the respective cast areas held with the fingers of the right hand.

During lateral movement, the right thumb tip depresses the side of the cast indicated by an arrow ①, while the other fingers grip the upper member of the articulator. When the shaft protrudes into the balancing side, a disocclusion of the condylar head and the shaft sheath takes place on the working side, as indicated by an arrow ②. If the anterior pin is moved alone with the fingertips, the Bennet movement cannot be correctly estimated.

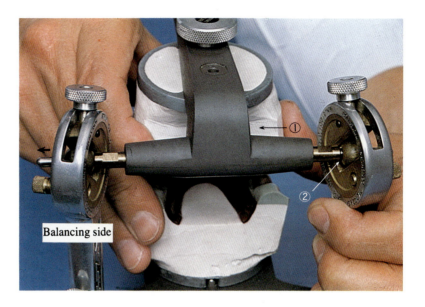

Lateral movement should be determined from the dentist's information, and necessary adjustments made after checking the occlusal contacts of the anterior teeth with contact ribbon. The angle of the incisal table is left at 0° on the sagittal plane.

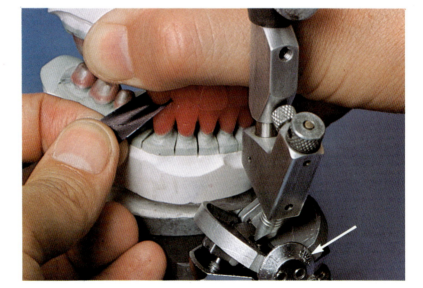

An adjustment of the maxillary canine is made on the working side in lateral excursion.

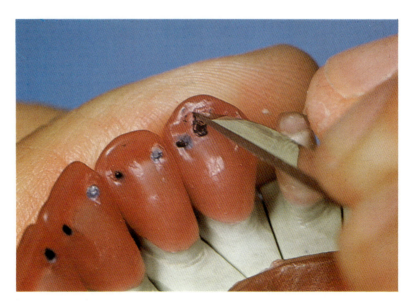

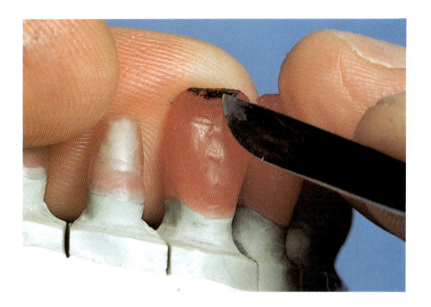

The lateral contact area of the working surface on the cusp of the mandibular canine is adjusted to form a line. This adjustment of the cusp tip is made with reference to the cuspal inclines of the working side.

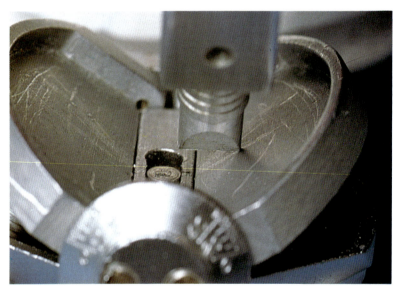

When the right lateral movement is performed properly, the angulations of the lateral wing of the adjustable incisal table and the tip of the anterior pin are in harmony with the excursion movements.

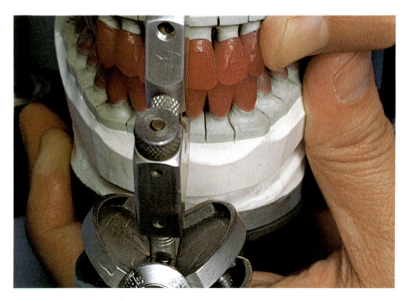

As on the right side, the left anterior guidance is similarly adjusted during a lateral movement. The right thumb tip is placed against the canine and the side of the model, while the other four fingers hold the upper member from above. The left thumb serves as a support for the right thumb, whose movement is controlled by the former.

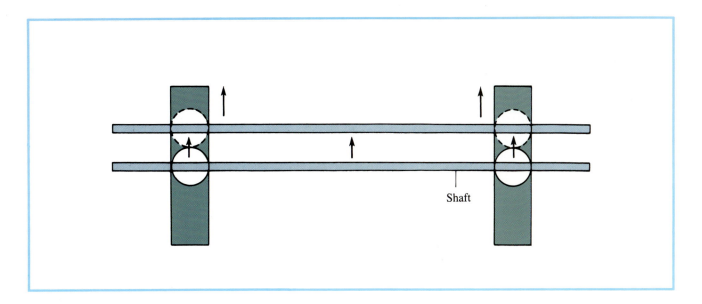

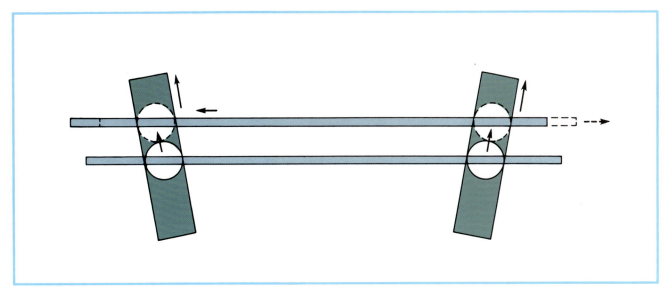

Unless the right and left movement angles are set at 0° in the forward movement, the shaft will be unstable and it is difficult to obtain the movement of a straight line pattern. When a lateral condylar angle is given, the distance between the condylar heads tends to become widened, as shown in this illustration.

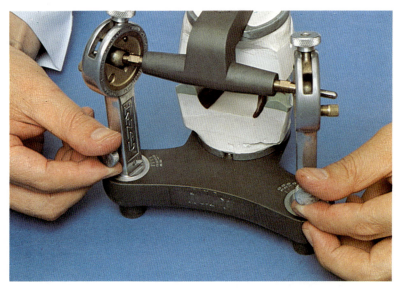

Therefore, the right and left lateral condylar angles are set at 0° in a forward movement.

141

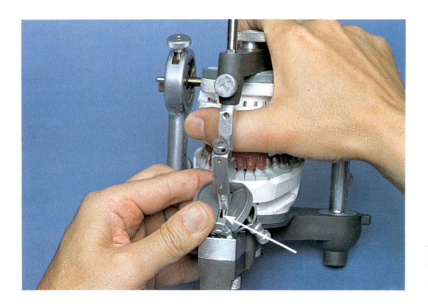

The anterior guidance table must be adjusted according to the information arrived at from diagnostic casts supplied by the dentist. The Long Centric Freedom table must be adjusted in harmony with the anterior pin.

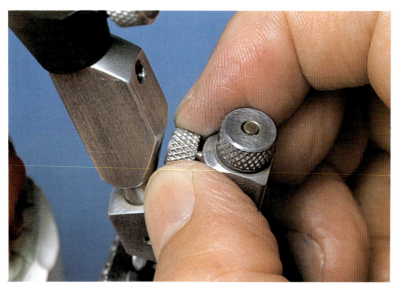

The adjustable anterior pin facilitates vertical adjustment whenever necessary.

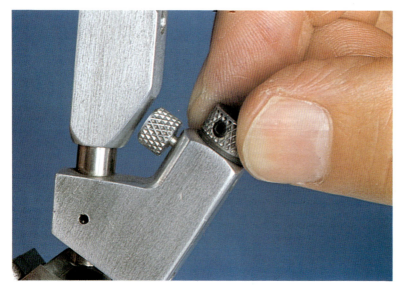

The adjustable anterior pin also makes it possible to maintain the exact position of the pin on the anterior table.

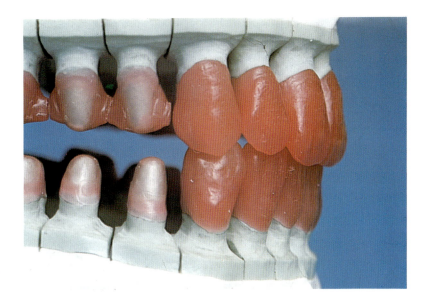

In this case, the use of the adjustable anterior pin facilitates establishment of the original vertical dimension.

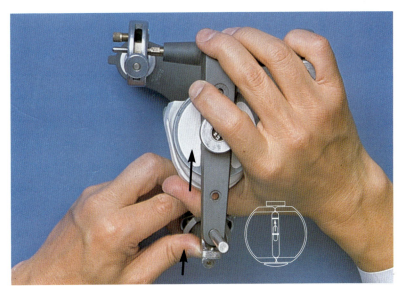

In order to secure straight protrusive movement, the adjustable anterior pin is guided along the center rail. Proper finger manipulation is essential for the straight movement.

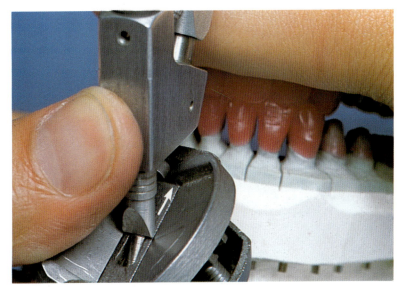

This close-up demonstrates proper digital manipulation during this movement: as the operator pushes the anterior pin back with his left thumb, he supports the maxillary planning wax crowns with the inside of his right thumb.

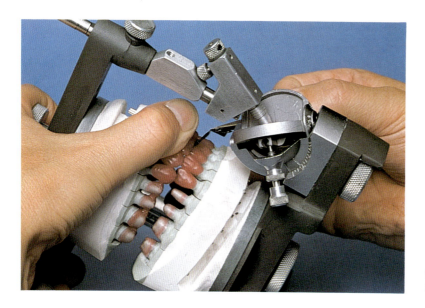

The lateral wings of the adjustable incisal table are raised steeply in order to secure straight protrusive movement.

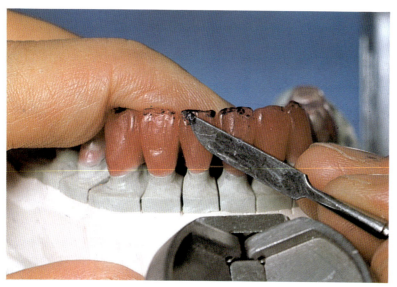

The working surfaces of the mandibular incisors are adjusted to correspond with the lingual inclines of the opposing teeth.

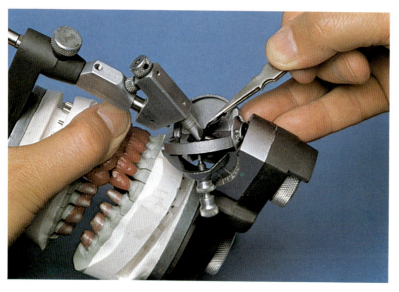

After completed straight protrusive adjustment, lateral protrusive movement is performed.

The wax crowns of the upper and lower anterior teeth after the completed anterior guidance procedure.

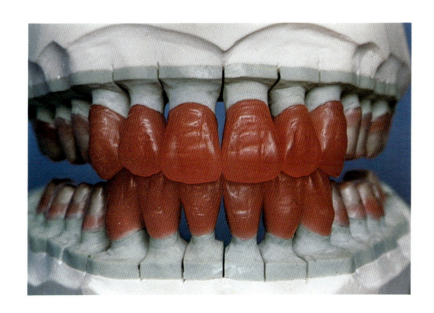

With protrusive movement, the relationship of the molar inclination (P_3) to the sagittal condylar angle (C_3) and the anterior guidance angle (A_3) can be mathematically expressed as follows:

$$P_3 = \frac{A_3 + C_3}{2} \dotso \text{(iii)}$$

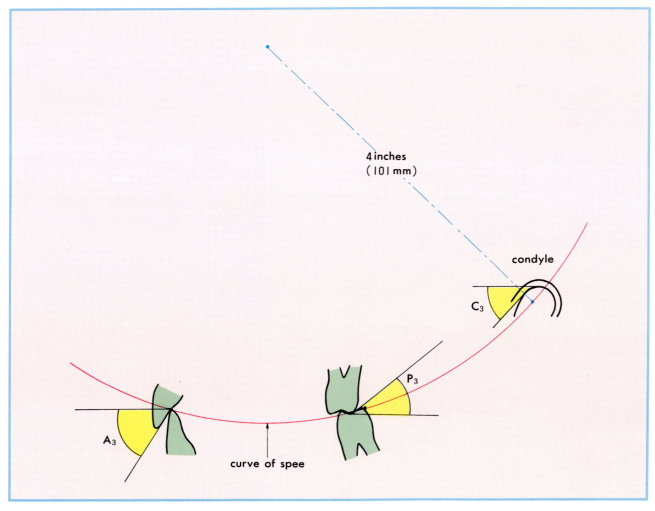

4 inches
(101 mm)

condyle

C_3

P_3

A_3

curve of spee

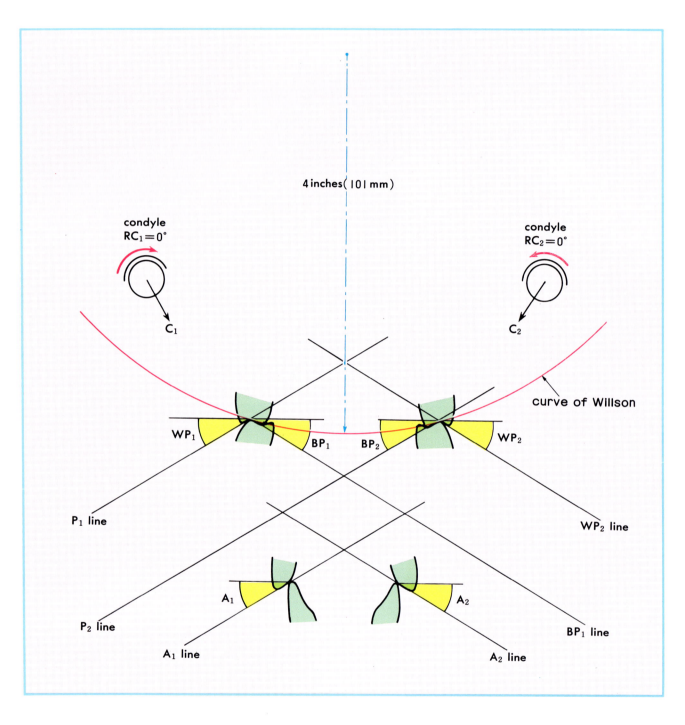

A schematic illustration of the condylar movement and the anterior guidance expressed in form of equations.

$$WP_1 = \frac{A_1 + RC_1(=0°)}{2} \ . \ . \ . \ . \ (i)$$

$$BP_2 = \frac{A_1 + C_2}{2} \ . \ . \ . \ . \ (ii)$$

$$BP_1 = \frac{A_2 + C_1}{2} \ . \ . \ . \ . \ (iv)$$

$$WP_2 = \frac{A_2 + RC_2(=0°)}{2} \ . \ . \ . \ . \ (v)$$

ANTERIOR GUIDANCE: DEFINITION

Anterior guidance plays an important part in the wax-up of the maxillary and mandibular crowns. We must know the relationship between the anterior guidance angle and the cuspal inclinations in the molar region. The numerical values for those are derived from the following set of equations:

1. The inclination on the working side of molar WP_1, between the canine and the temporomandibular joint, equals the lateral movement:

$$WP_1 = \frac{A_1 + RC_1(=0°)}{2} \quad \ldots \ldots \text{ (i)}$$

where

A_1 = The anterior guidance angle for the canine on the working side in the right lateral movement

RC_1 = The rotation of the condyle on the right working side ($=0°$)

The value obtained from this equation is applied in the concept of group function. The width of the contact area and the curvatures of the buccal cusps can also be roughly determined from the same numerical value.

2. The inclination of the molars (BP_2) on the balancing side between the canine and the temporomandibular joint equals the right lateral movement:

$$BP_2 = \frac{A_1 + C_2}{2} \quad \ldots \ldots \text{ (ii)}$$

where

C_2 = The condylar angle on the left balancing side

In order to avoid occlusal contacts between the molars on the balancing side, the numerical value should not exceed the angulations of the inner inclines of the molars.

3. The inclination of the sagittal plane of the molar (P_3) between the canine and temporomandibular joint equals:

$$P_3 = \frac{A_3 + C_3}{2} \quad \ldots \ldots \text{ (iii)}$$

where

A_3 = The anterior guidance angle for the canine in the protrusive movement

C_3 = The sagittal condylar angle

From these considerations, it is evident that construction of the anterior guidances enables us to analyze the relationships of various mandibular movements and occlusal surfaces in a geometrical manner. The condyles within the temporomandibular fossa show a complicated three-dimensional movement which greatly influences the contours of the occlusal surfaces. Limitations of the condylar movement can cause a host of problems, especially involving the molar region.

Numerical values derived from the equations above represent some standard values which are applied when using a fully adjustable articulator, and when using the F.G.P. technique and the various electronic apparatuses available to us now.

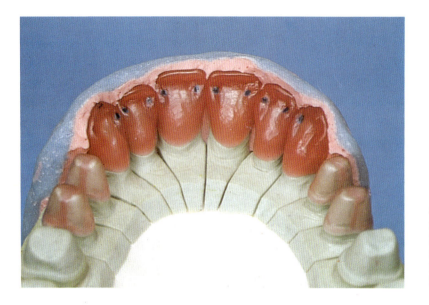

3.3.4 SILICONE INDEX CORE AND RESIN CANINE DESIGN

After the anterior guidances are set for the maxillary and mandibular anterior teeth, the final crown contour is waxed up. At this stage, silicone molds are made of the maxillary and mandibular anterior teeth, including both the labial and the cervical areas.

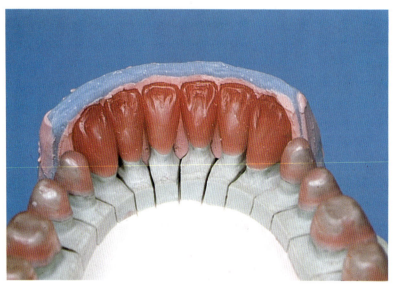

This core will serve as an index for subsequent porcelain construction. See Volume II, Ch. 7. A silicone index is made from the maxillary anterior teeth.

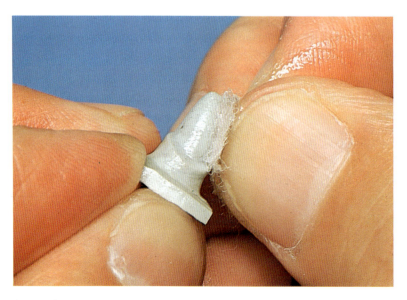

This will serve as a basis for the resin canines during the subsequent stages of this procedure. In order to maintain the vertical dimension and to preserve accurate records of the lateral movements, the maxillary and mandibular canine wax patterns are replaced with resin crowns. The canine die is coated with a separator such as vaseline.

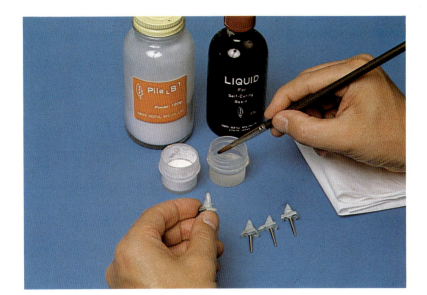

The canine pattern is made with an appropriate amount of chemically polymerizing acrylic resin, which is applied carefully with a brush onto the die.

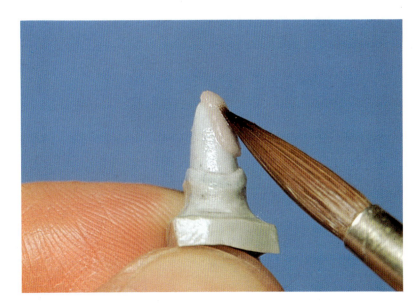

When the resin has set, the pattern is removed from the die.

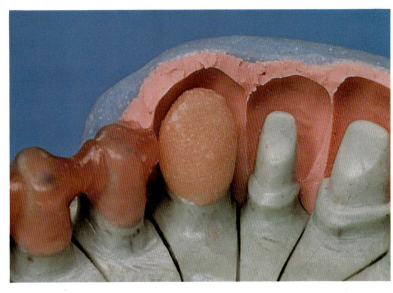

Now the silicone index is placed over the die. This will help us estimate the amount of resin still needed to arrive at the former size of the wax pattern.

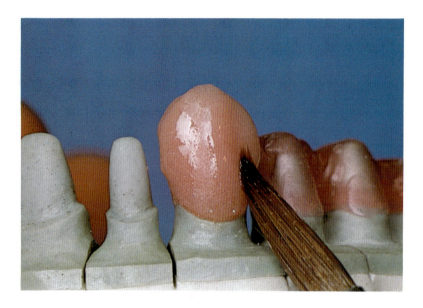

By adding more resin to the pattern the crown form is roughly completed. If needed, more resin is added onto the labial surface of the crown.

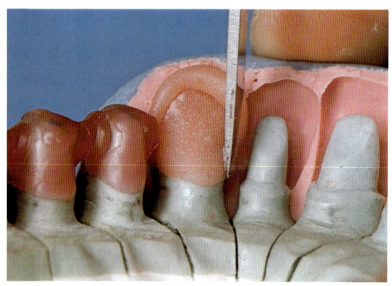

The silicone index is replaced on the pattern. Any resin excess is cut off with the carving knife.

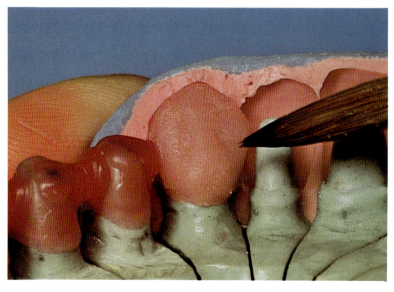

The lingual contour is shaped after adding more resin. For the maxillary anterior teeth, an allowance must be made for adjustments in lateral movement.

After the maxillary and mandibular resin crowns are manufactured, right and left lateral movements are confirmed and adjustments made, based on anterior guidance information registered with the anterior guidance table.

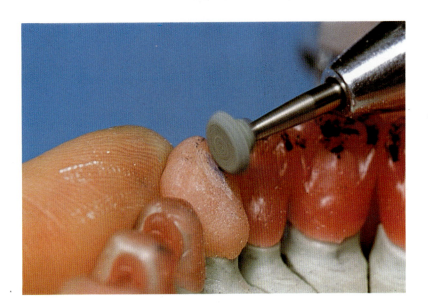

The data recorded on the contact ribbon is used for adjustments of the inclines of the maxillary canines on the working side.

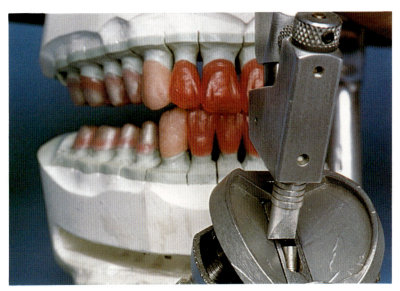

The same process is repeated on the opposite side. Again, information gained from the registrations at the anterior guidance table is utilized.

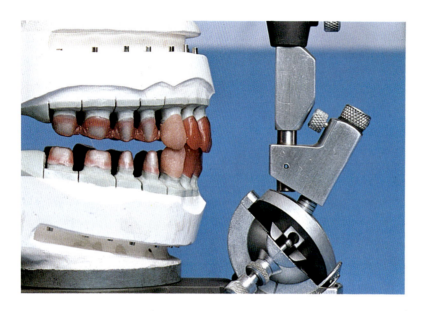

Completed right maxillary and mandibular canine resin crowns.

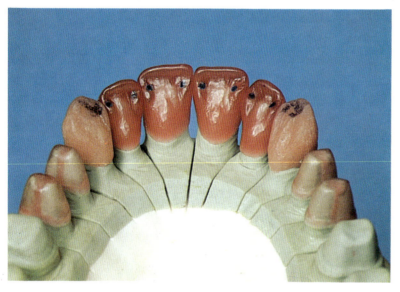

The resin canine crowns are strong enough to withstand the impact of lateral movements, thus protecting the anterior guidances of the maxillary and mandibular wax crowns from injury.

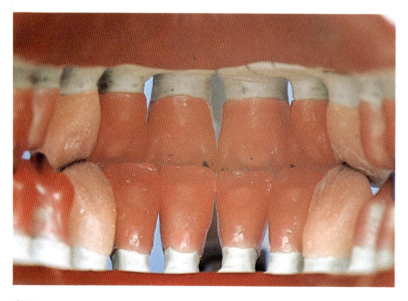

The vertical dimension is also stabilized through the resin crown.

3.3.5 DESIGN OF THE MOLAR WAX PATTERN (SKELETAL TECHNIQUE AND THREE DIMENSIONAL WAXING TECHNIQUE)

Goals:
1. Occlusal contact of as many teeth as possible in centric relation occlusion.
2. Direction of occlusal loading parallel to the long axis of the tooth.
3. During the protrusive movement, as many anterior teeth as possible make contact in group function. No occlusal contact between posterior teeth in a protrusive movement.
4. During lateral movements, the canines, along with the posterior teeth, make contact on the working side, never on the balancing side.

In the P.M.S. system (named after Pankey, Mann and Schuyler), an arch with a radius of 4 inches is drawn, contacting the cusp tip of the mandibular canine and the disto-buccal cusp of the 2nd molar; another arch, also 4 inches in radius, is used as the Spee curve. (It becomes evident that the so-called Spee's curve in the P.M.S. system differs somewhat from the original curve introduced by Spee in 1890. When quoting Spee's curve in this publicaton we will follow the usage of Pankey, Mann and Schuyler.)

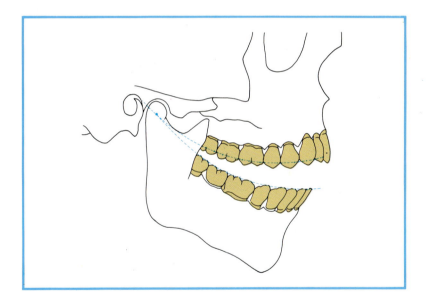

Both Spee's curve and Wilson's curve are illustrated here. One objective of the P.M.S. system is to ideally position all the teeth along these curves in occlusal contact and centric relation. The 4-inch radius is derived from the theory of Monson's sphere (illustration: courtesy from Monson, G.S., 1920).

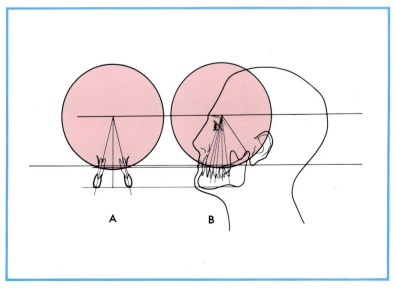

A   B

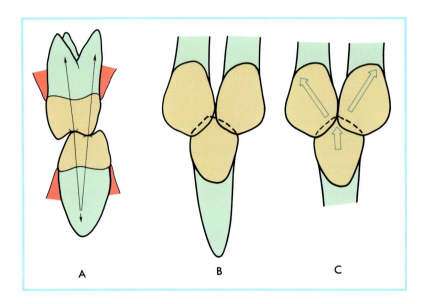

As stated above, one important goal is to channel the direction of the occlusal forces along the long axis of the tooth. The interdigitation of the cusp into the fossa as in A is necessary, but at the same time, it is essential that the buccal cusp tips of the mandibular teeth come into contact with the cusp ridges of the maxillary teeth, as in B. If contact is made as in C, the tooth tends to exert lateral pressure onto two opposing teeth during mastication and food particles are directed into the proximal embrasures.

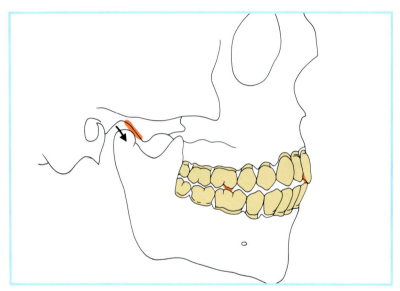

During protrusive movement, the anterior teeth alone are brought into occlusal contact, whereas the molars must never make contact. In order to accomplish this, the cuspal inclination angle should not be more acute than absolutely necessary.

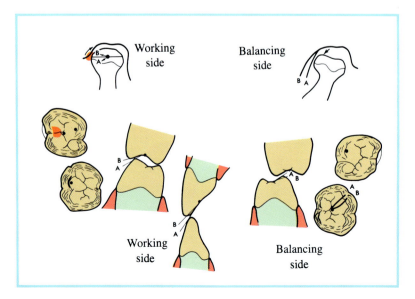

During lateral movement, the canines on the working side are brought into group function with due consideration of the curves of Spee and Wilson, in harmony with the condylar inclines and the anterior guidances. During lateral movement, the buccal cusp ridges of the mandibular teeth on the working side are in occlusal contact, determined by the anterior guidances and the condylar movements.

The diagnostic wax patterns for the mandibular molars are obtained in a manner similar to that used in the diagnostic wax-up of the anterior teeth. The procedure consists of the following six steps:

1) Placement of wax rods on the mandibular buccal cusp ridges.
2) Placement of wax rods on the maxillary lingual cusp ridges.
3) Waxing up the buccal cusps of the maxillary molars.
4) Reinforcement of the wax rods ①.
5) Reinforcement of the wax rods ②.
6) Removal of the ends of the wax rods ① and ②.

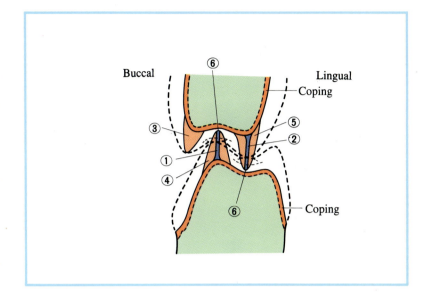

To begin, the wax rods are placed onto the respective buccal cusps to determine the buccal occlusal points.

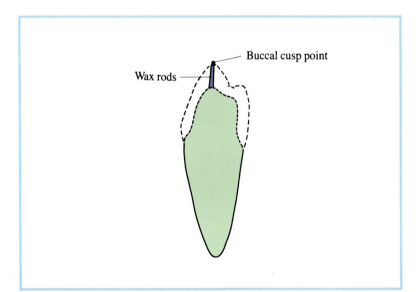

The patterns of the respective maxillary molars are waxed together buccolingually, and the mandibular molars are notched with a carving knife to indicate the areas for positioning of the wax rods. This procedure is in line with the requirement of directing occlusal loading aong the long axes of teeth.

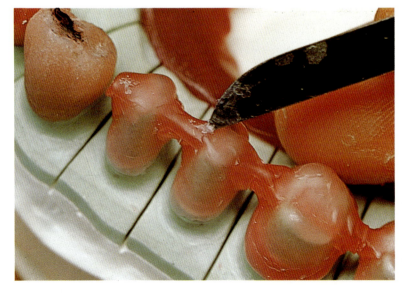

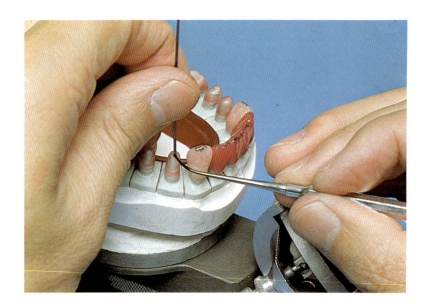

0.7mm thick wax rods are placed into the positions already marked on the mandibular buccal cusps of the premolars. The wax rods are slightly heated and placed in position with a M.K. instrument.

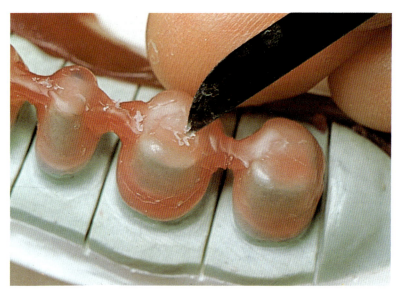

The maxillary molars are similarly marked. Here the best result is obtained when the occlusal contact line is marked along the central fossae.

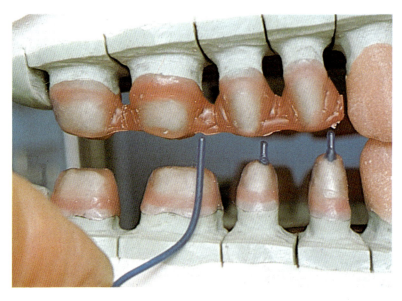

The positions for the wax rods are confirmed on the buccal cusps of the maxillary first molars by referring to the marks previously registered.

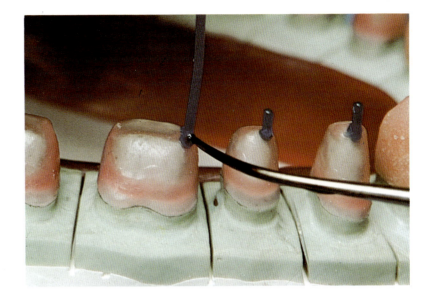

The wax rods are placed on the buccal cusps of the mandibular first molar.

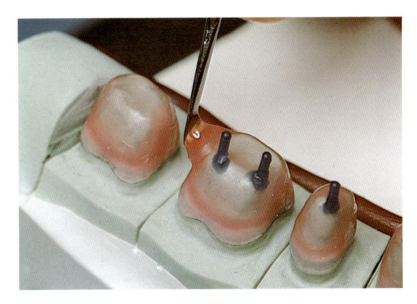

If placement of the wax rods poses a problem, we can add some inlay wax onto the pattern in order to facilitate the procedure.

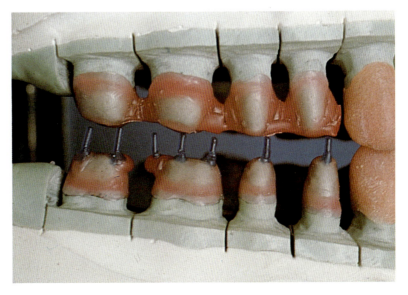

Wax rods have been implanted on all buccal cusps of the mandibular molars. Occasionally, the wax rods must be reinforced with additional wax at their base.

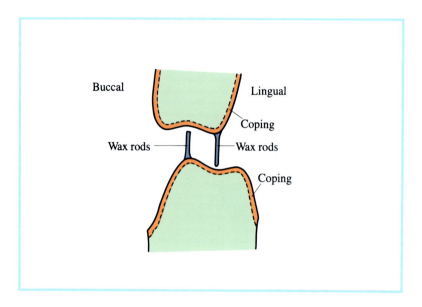

The next step is the placement of the wax rods on the maxillary lingual cusps to establish centric occlusion points. Lengths are adjusted to avoid contact with the patterns of the opposing teeth.

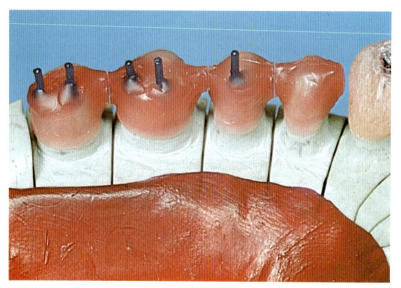

The wax rods are placed on the maxillary lingual cusps, excluding the cusps of the first premolars. For convenience's sake the procedure is completed by working on individual teeth and their respective opponents one at a time. Proximal relationships are checked frequently.

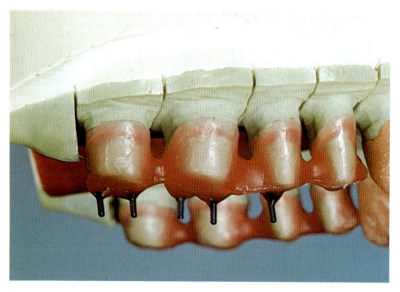

A buccal view of the maxillary posterior teeth with the wax rods implanted. The small marks seen on the proximal areas indicate future contact areas.

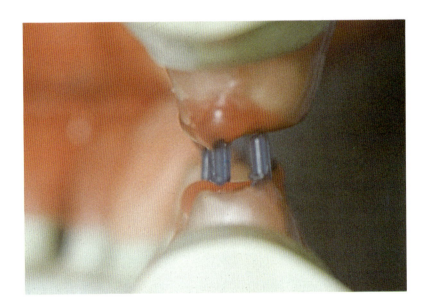

The occlusal relationships of the mandibular buccal and maxillary lingual cusps are examined closely.

A distal view of the same. The distance between the buccal and lingual cusps must account for 55 to 60% of crown width.

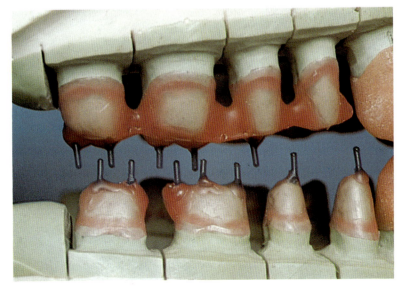

With the wax rods on the maxillary and mandibular posterior teeth, the molar wax patterns are examined for occlusal clearance during lateral movement. This confirmation of occlusal molar relationships is an important feature of the diagnostic **three-dimensional wax up.**

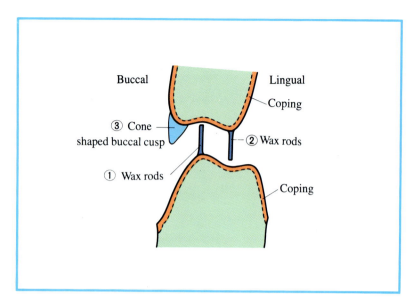

Buccal   Lingual
                          Coping
③ Cone
shaped buccal cusp   ② Wax rods
① Wax rods
                          Coping

During the next step, the buccal cusps of the maxillary molars are waxed up in a cone shape.

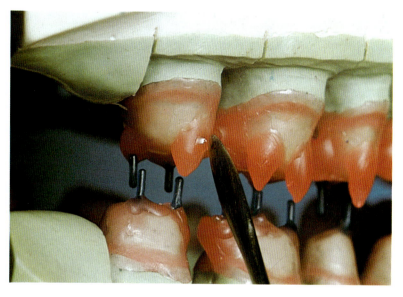

Remember that preparation of the wax rods aids in determining the relative positions of the mandibular wax rods and the maxillary buccal cusps during lateral movements.

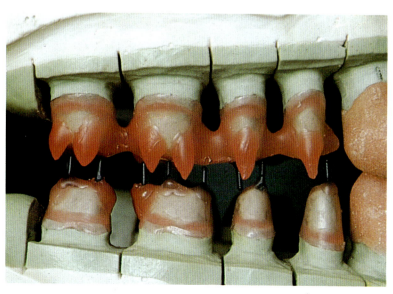

A buccal view of the prepared wax rods in centric relation occlusion.

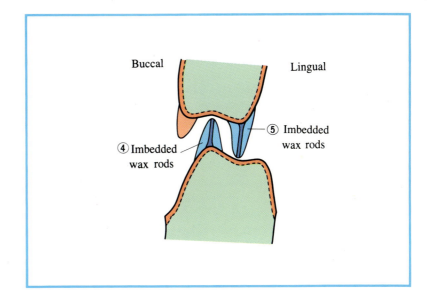

A lateral movement is effected on the working side in order to examine the maxillary and mandibular wax rods and the maxillary buccal cusps for lateral contacts and for clearance of the wax rods during this movement.

Buccal   Lingual

⑤ Imbedded
wax rods

④ Imbedded
wax rods

From this, it is evident that the positions of the maxillary molars are determined by the opposing mandibular teeth. Thus we are able to plan the rough outlines of the maxillary molars.

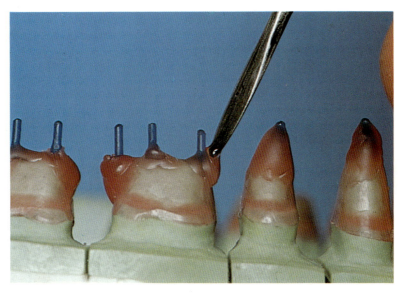

The wax rods are reinforced with inlay wax at their bases. When reinforcing the wax rods, care must be taken not to melt them. The color-coded waxes (blue for rods, pink for inlay wax) help us to distinguish between the different structures, and to avoid errors in waxing.

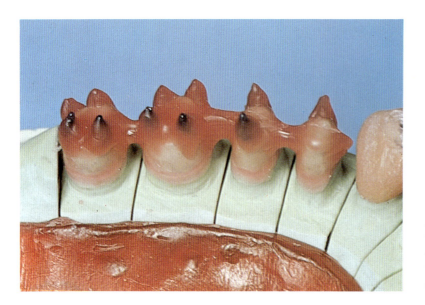

A lingual view of the occlusal surfaces of the maxillary molars after the wax rods have been reinforced. The diagnostic wax-up for the maxillary crowns is completed as a preliminary measure for the subsequent wax-up of the mandibular molars.

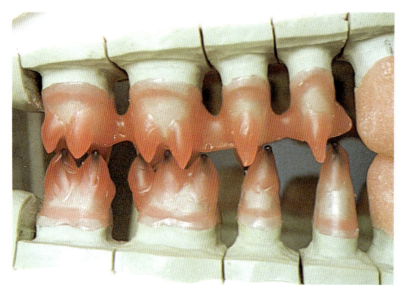

The maxillary and mandibular molars (with reinforced wax rods) are brought into occlusal contact.

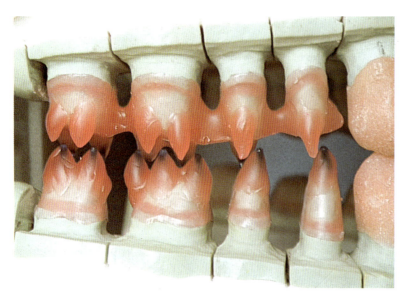

During lateral movement on the working side, the relationship between the buccal cusps of the mandibular premolars and the inclinations of the maxillary premolars can be clearly examined.

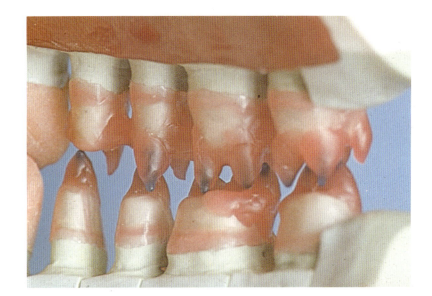

Final confirmation during lateral movement on the balancing side.

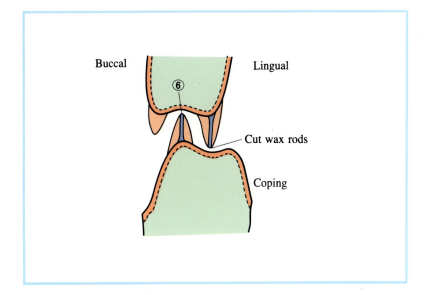

Buccal

Lingual

⑥

Cut wax rods

Coping

The tips of the wax rods are left somewhat longer than the length of the wax cusp tips.

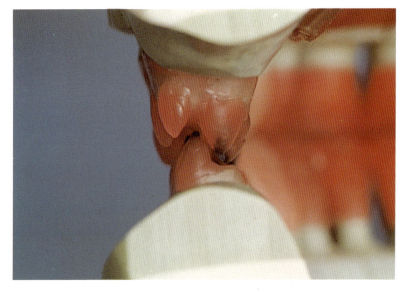

The tips of the wax rods have been cut off. For convenience, it may be wise to eliminate the maxillary buccal cusps during the establishment of the occlusal surfaces.

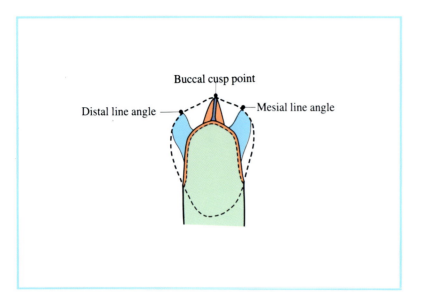

Buccal cusp point

Distal line angle — — Mesial line angle

At this stage, all buccal cusp tips of the posterior teeth (orange shaded area) are complete.

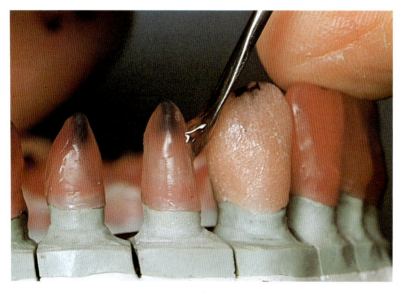

Now the mesial and distal line angle points are established on the mandibular first premolar, while frequently checking occlusal relation with the opposing teeth.

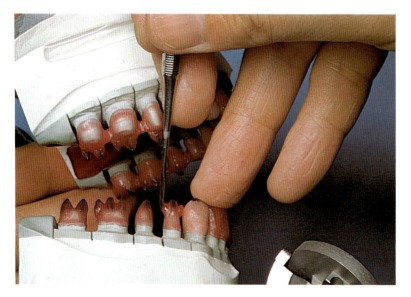

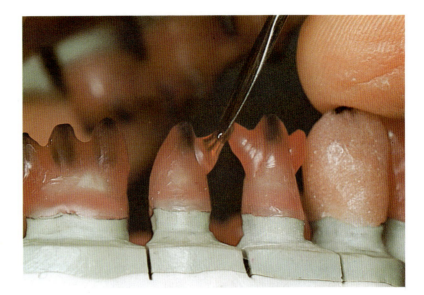

The mesial line angle is now waxed up for the mandibular second premolar.

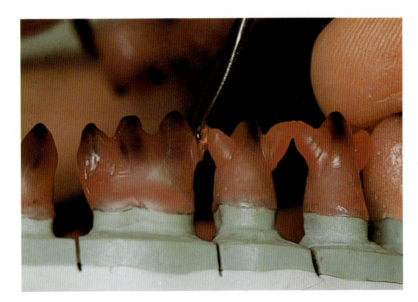

Similarly, the mesial line angle point on the mandibular first molar is waxed up and, as always, the temperature of the wax must be carefully controlled in order to avoid any distortion of the line angles of the adjacent teeth.

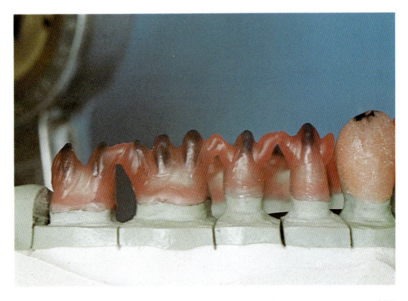

The mesiodistal line angle points of the mandibular molars have now been established. The mesiodistal line angle points of the second molar were previously established.

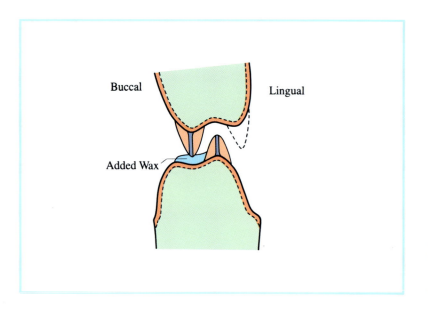

Buccal   Lingual

Added Wax

When the mesiodistal line angles of the mandibular molar are waxed up, the space between the tips of the maxillary wax rods and the occlusal surface of the mandibular pattern is examined.

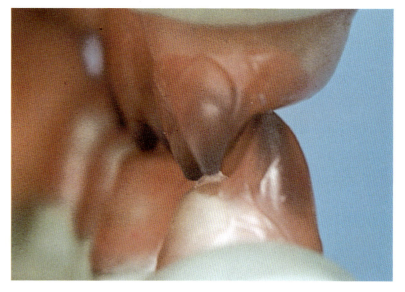

Now a small amount of wax is added to the mandibular pattern. The maxillary and mandibular teeth are brought into occlusal contact, and the markings of the maxillary lingual cusp tips are registered.

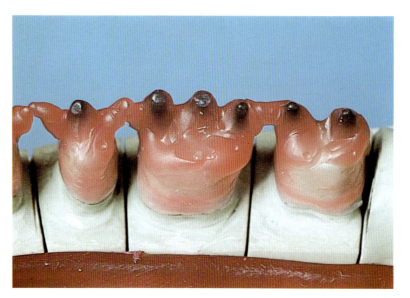

The indentations thus obtained will serve as fossa points on the mandibular molars and will be used during the subsequent fabrication of wax patterns.

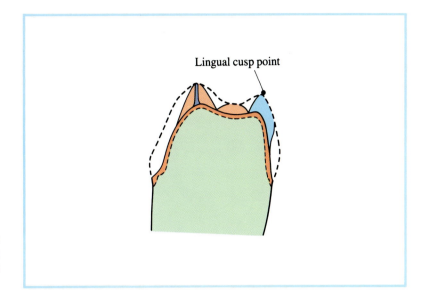

Lingual cusp point

The lingual cusp tips of the mandibular molars are waxed up, taking in consideration the three planes that constitute the crown contour.

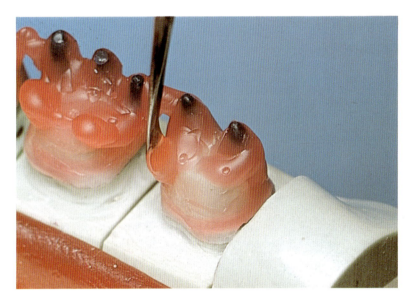

The lingual cusp tips of the mandibular second molar are waxed up. Here we must avoid letting any wax flow into the central fossa dot. The occlusal relationship with the teeth of the opposing arch must be checked frequently.

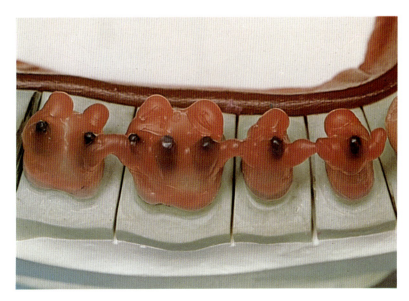

The lingual cusp tips have been established on the mandibular molars. At this stage, it is possible to estimate final crown contour.

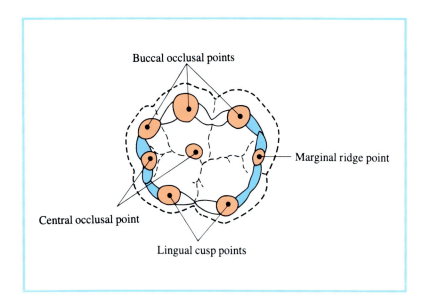

Buccal occlusal points

Marginal ridge point

Central occlusal point

Lingual cusp points

An outline of the mandibular occlusal surface is established by building up the cusp ridges.

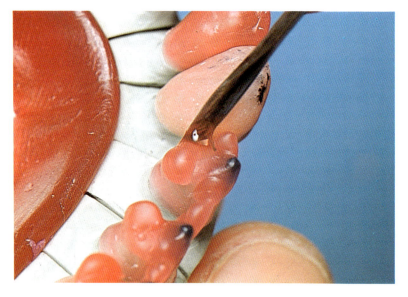

The mesial cusp ridges are waxed up on the mandibular first premolar.

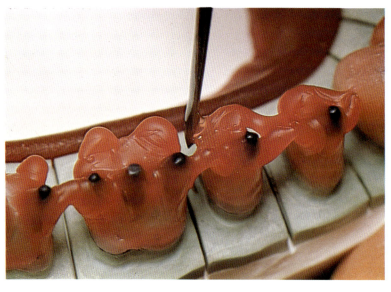

The distal cusp ridges of the mandibular second premolar are built up.

The mesial cusp ridges of the mandibular first molar are built up, avoiding any excess accumulation around the central occlusal point (indicated by the indentation of the maxillary lingual cusp tip).

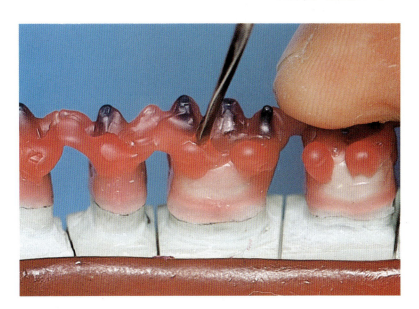

Close-up view of the lingual wax up.

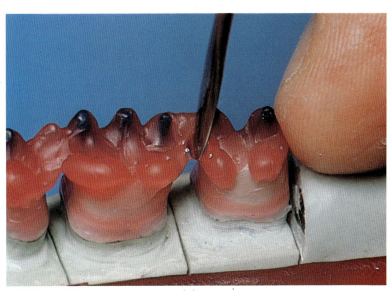

The lingual cusp ridges are similarly built up on the mandibular second molar.

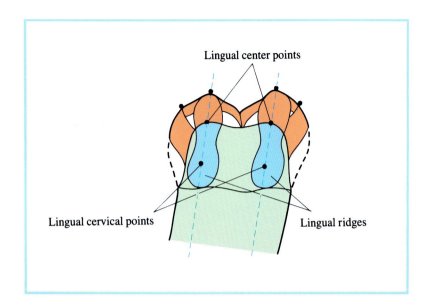

Lingual center points

Lingual cervical points

Lingual ridges

The lingual ridges are built up to join the cusps and the gingival third of the lingual surface. Ridges and grooves are constructed with reference to root contour.

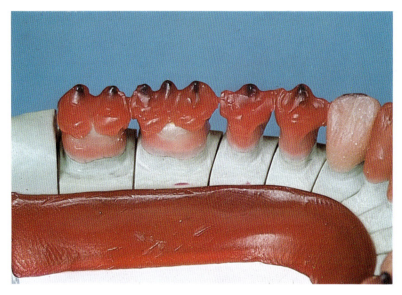

From this angle, it is possible to see a continuity between the buccal cusps, buccal cusp ridges, lingual cusps, lingual cusp ridges and the roots of the first and second premolars.

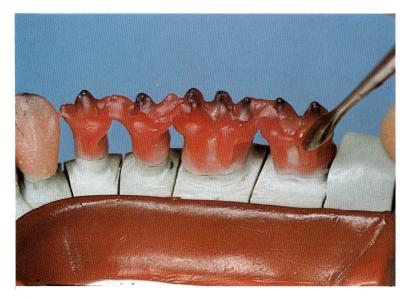

The first and second mandibular molar ridges are built up on the mesiodistal lingual surfaces. By furnishing these mesiodistal lingual ridges, the form of the lingual grooves and continuity to the root surface are both accomplished.

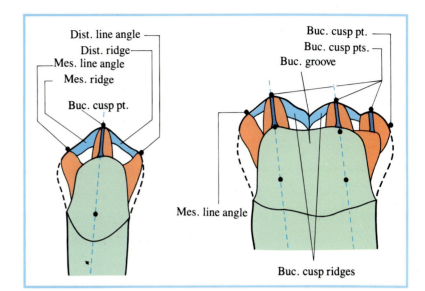

The mesiodistal line angle and buccal fossa point are joined through the mesial and distal cusp ridge of the mandibular first molar.

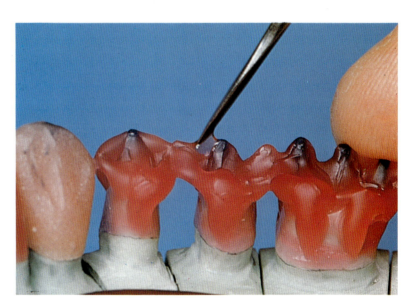

The same procedure is followed on the second premolar. As always, the proper amount and correct temperature of the wax is crucial.

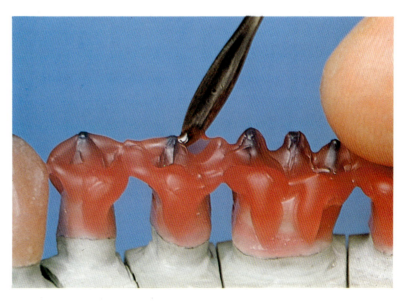

The distal line angle of the second premolar is joined to the buccal occlusal point on the distal cusp ridge.

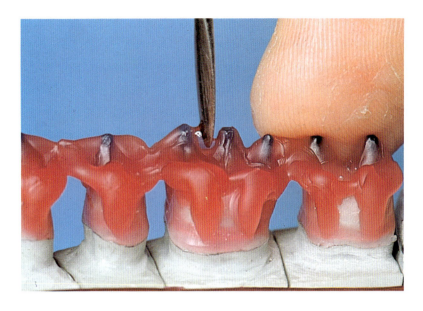

Similarly, the mesial line angle of the first molar and the buccal cusp tip are connected.

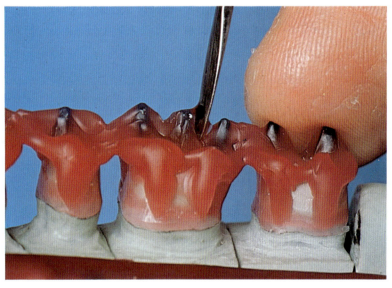

The distal marginal ridge of the mandibular first molar is already waxed when the distal line angle is established.

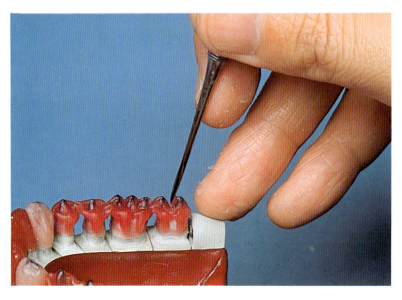

The mesial and distal buccal cusps and the distal cusp are waxed up. From these skeletons, the functional and anatomical outlines of crown contour can be established.

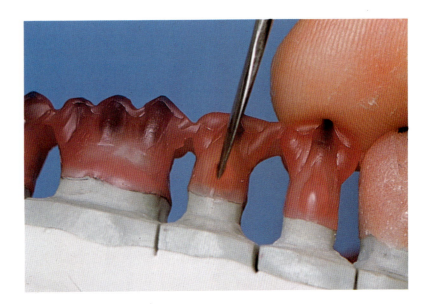

Here, the buccal cervical ridge is constructed on the mandibular first molar. Reference to a dental morphology atlas will facilitate this procedure.

Here the buccal cervical ridge is waxed on the mandibular second premolar. The buccal cervical ridge is basically on the same line as the buccal cervical point and the center of the root.

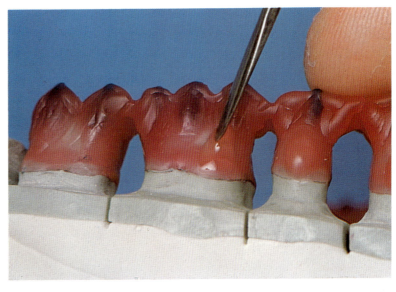

The mesial buccal cervical ridge is constructed on the mandibular first molar. Here we must keep in mind that the lines from the respective cusps should be aligned with the buccal cervical ridge.

173

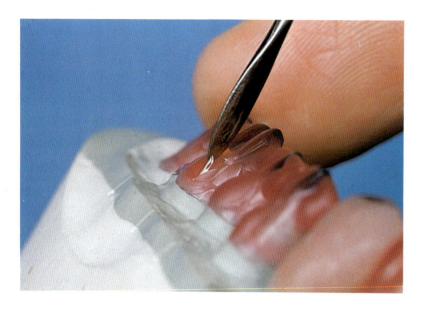

When forming the buccal cervical ridge, we must remember that crown contour is established in three planes. The height of contour and the most prominent part of the cervical ridge coincide.

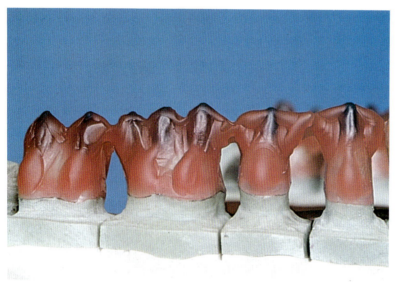

All buccal cervical ridges of the mandibular molars are completed.

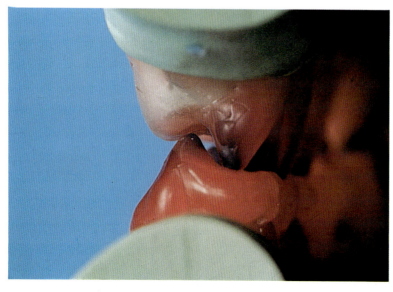

A distal view of the same. As the buccal cervical line is already prepared, the remaining two planes are added at a later time.

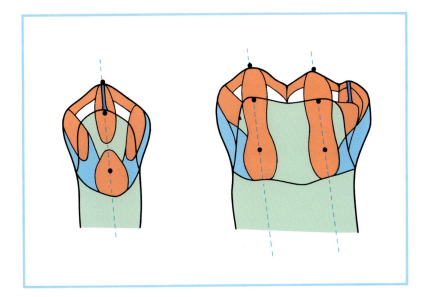

The space between the mesiodistal line angle and the buccal ridges is filled in.

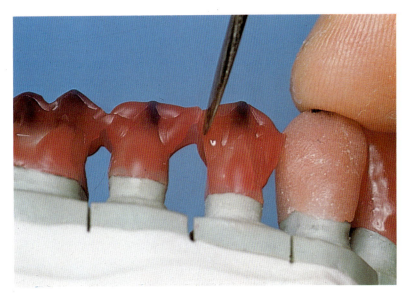

Observing the proximal relationship to adjacent teeth, the distal buccal ridge is constructed.

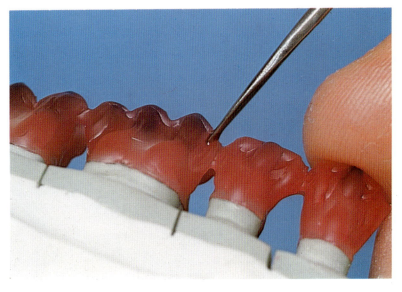

The mesial cusp ridge is waxed up on the mesiobuccal cusp of the first molar. The next step is the wax-up of the mesial and distal cusp ridges of the buccal cusps of the second molar.

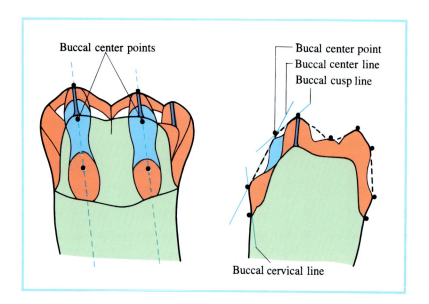

Buccal center points

Bucal center point
Buccal center line
Buccal cusp line

Buccal cervical line

Now the disto-buccal cusp is waxed up, followed by the buccal center line and the buccal cusp line.

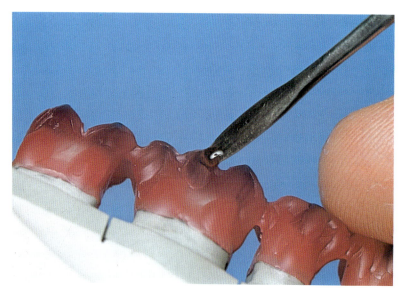

After the buccal cusp tip of the mandibular premolar is established, the distobuccal cusp tip of the first molar is waxed up.

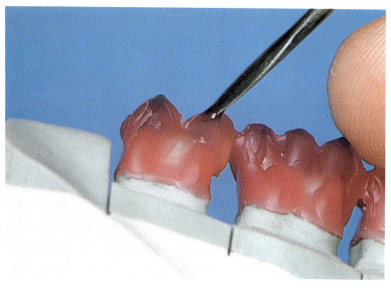

The same procedure is completed on the second molar. The buccal center ridge and the buccal cervical ridge are joined to form the cusp ridge.

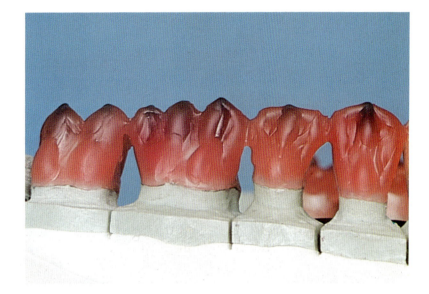

The buccal cusp tips of the mandibular molars are now completed, thus establishing all necessary landmark points. After connecting those areas, we are ready for the wax up of the crowns.

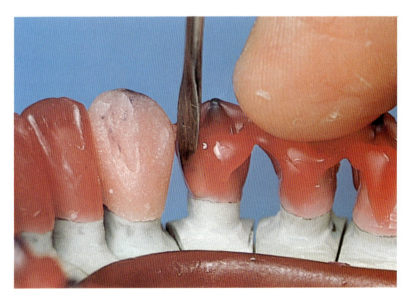

After the basic skeleton has been established, the remaining areas are filled in with wax.

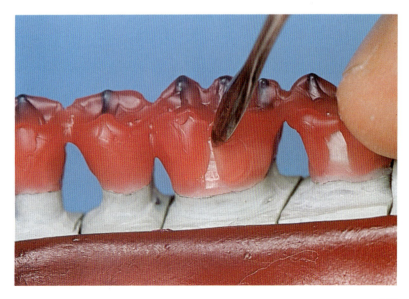

After the area between the mesial lingual cusp ridge and the marginal ridge of the mesiolingual cusp of the first molar is filled, the lingual groove is contoured. Again, it is important to carefully monitor the amount and temperature of the wax.

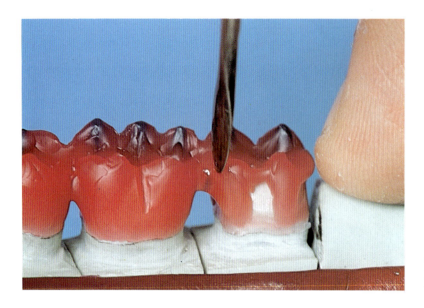

Next, the area between the distal cusp ridge of the distolingual cusp of the mandibular first molar and the marginal ridge is filled in with wax.

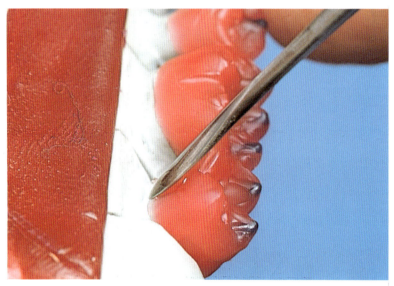

The wax-up is continued in the area between the lingual grooves and the lingual cervical portions for the same teeth. The three-dimensional contour is created by filling in the areas between these landmark points of wax.

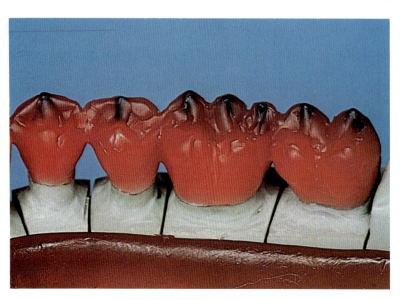

Using the above procedure, the lingual outline is obtained.

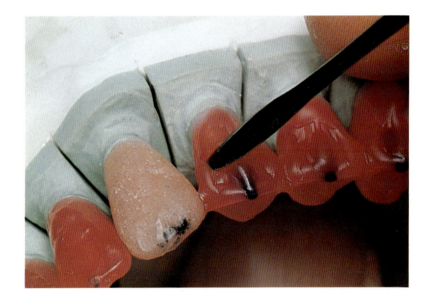

The landmark ridges on the buccal side are linked to each other, first mesially, then distally.

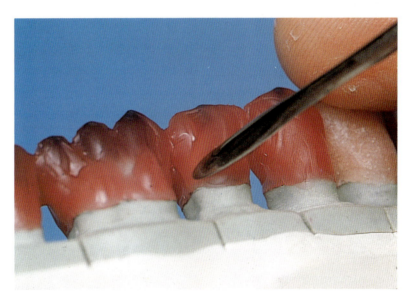

The same procedure is repeated for the second premolars.

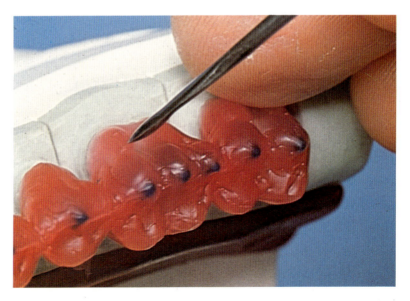

The same procedure is repeated in the molar area.

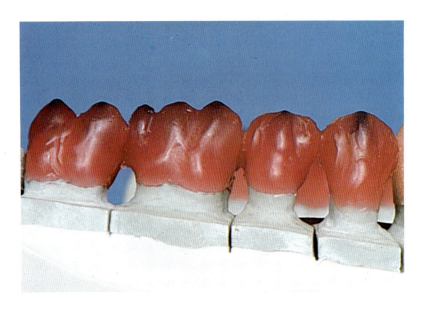

A buccal view of the right mandibular molar region, where the crown contours are built up. At this point, we do not carve the wax crowns.

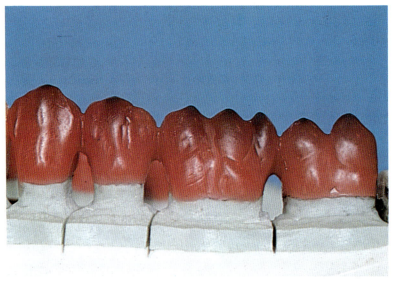

Another lateral view of the left mandibular region, where one can clearly observe various landmark points, ridges, and lines.

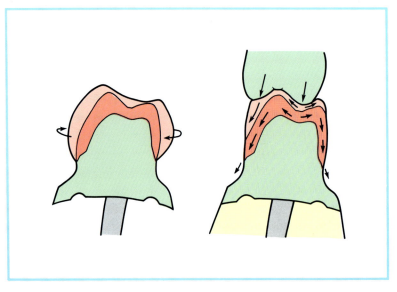

Proper wax control will affect the timing and success of any waxing procedure. Care is taken not to add more wax than necessary, so additional stress on the wax pattern can be avoided.

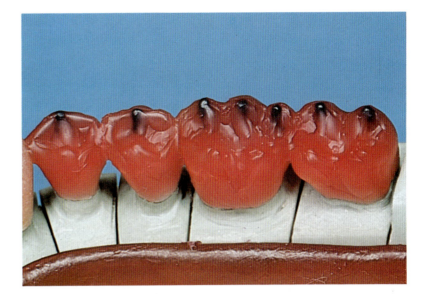

An occlusal view of the mandibular right molar region in with the crown contour. This region is built up using the skeletal technique.

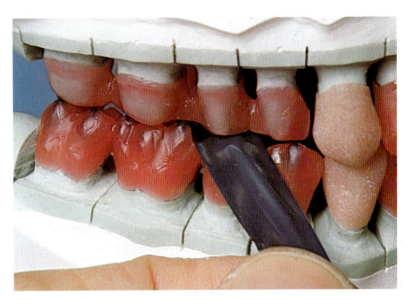

Occlusal markings, serving as centric occlusal stops, are best defined by using a contact ribbon.

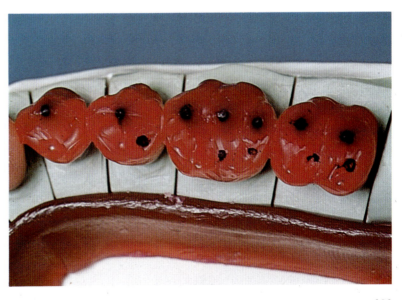

Occlusal marks thus registered can be clearly detected as centric occlusal stops on the occlusal surfaces opposite the maxillary lingual cusps.

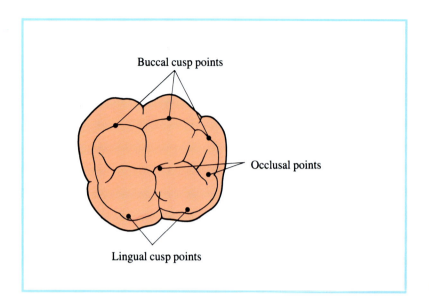

Buccal cusp points

Occlusal points

Lingual cusp points

A diagram of various landmark points essential for the wax up of the crown contours.

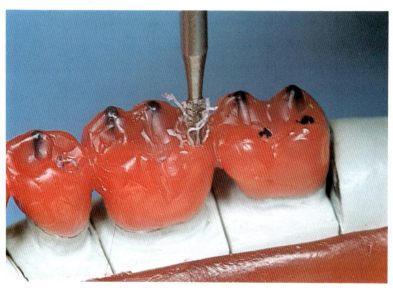

As described previously, holes are drilled into the occlusal stops with a bur of a diameter of 0.8 to 1.0mm. The depth of the holes does not extend to the die.

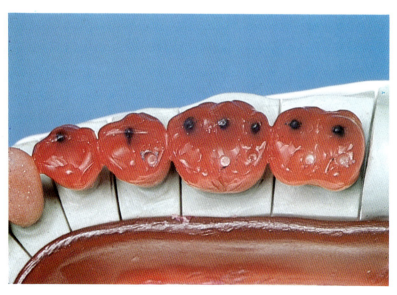

Holes with a diameter of 1.0mm are drilled into all centric occlusal stops on the right molar region.

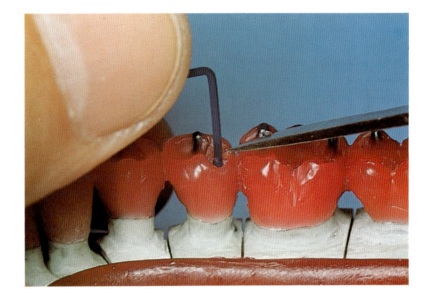

Wax rods are then placed into the prepared holes in the same manner as previously described.

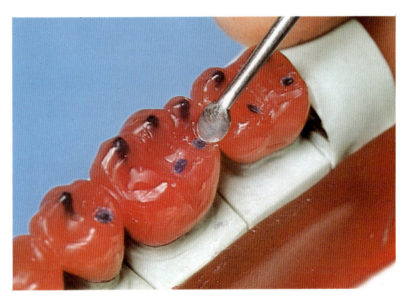

Any excess (of the wax rods) is cut off with a discoid carver.

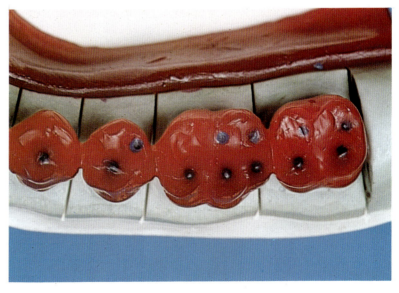

An occlusal view of the left molar region.

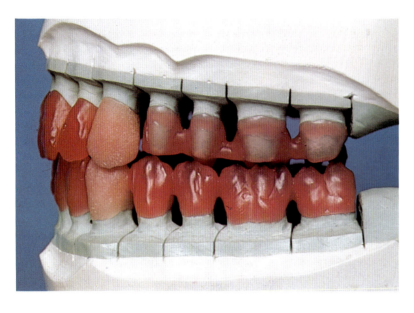

A buccal view of the left molar region.

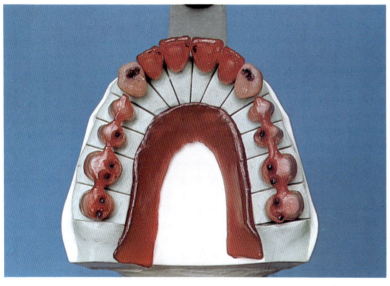

An occlusal view of the molar region with the anterior planning wax ups, the resin canines, and the maxillary lingual cusps.

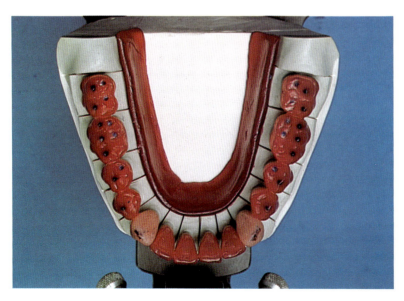

An occlusal view of the wax ups with the anterior planning wax ups, the resin canines, and the respective occlusal stops completed.

3.3.6. ESTABLISHING THE OCCLUSAL PLANE

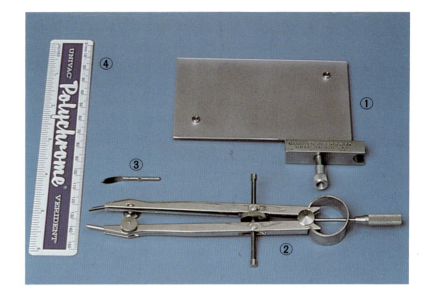

The occlusal planes of the mandibular molars (curves of Spee and Wilson) are established with the Broadlic occlusal plane analyzer (Hanau model 145-1), which consists of the following components:
① Flag
② Compasses
③ Cutting knife
④ Scale (in inches and centimeters)

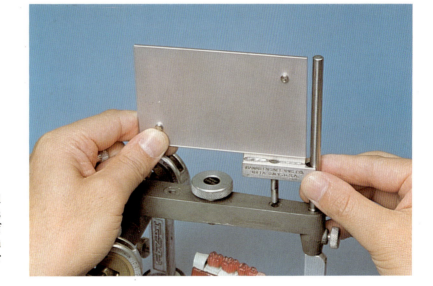

A plastic sheet is placed on the flag and kept in position with a screw. The flag is mounted on the articulator. Any type of Hanau articulator can be used in conjunction with the flag. Here, the Hanau articulator 145-2 is used.

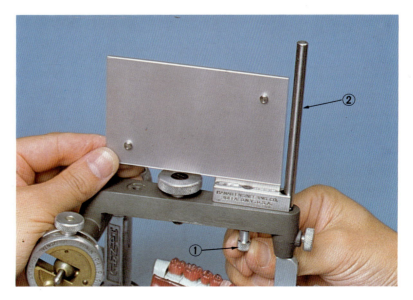

The flag is firmly fastened to the upper member with a screw and an extension pin.

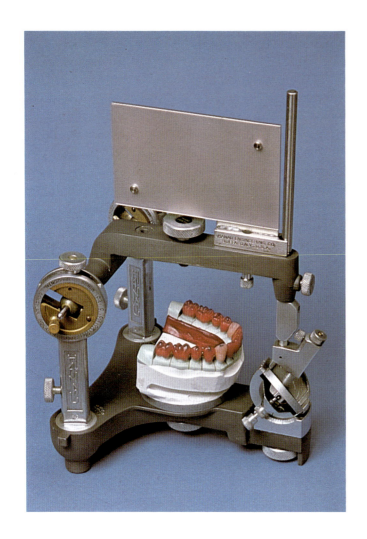

This illustration shows the flag mounted on the articulator.

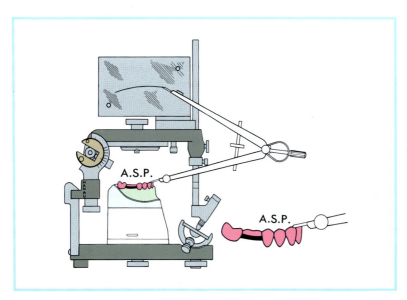

A.S.P.

A.S.P.

An A.S.P. (anterior survey point) is obtained somewhere between the canine cusp tip and the distal line angle. With the A.S.P. as the center, an arch with a radius of 4 inches is scribed on the plastic sheet (illustration courtesy of the P.M.S. Manual). In this procedure, the nearer the A.S.P. position is to the distal line angle (from the canine cusp tip), the lower the height of that occlusal surface. Therefore, the A.S.P. serves as a reference for the length of the crown and its relation to the maxillary molars.

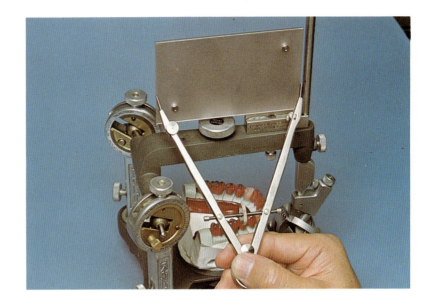

The A.S.P. arch, which has a radius of 4 inches and is registered on the plastic sheet attached to the flag, can be directly transferred to the compasses as shown.

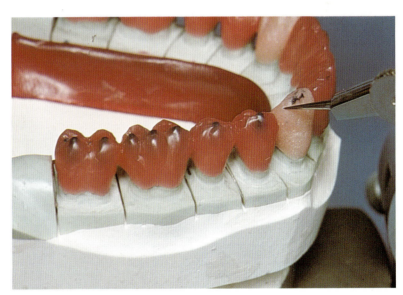

The A.S.P. is obtained on the canine cusp tip, which has important bearings on the setup of the occlusal mandibular molar surfaces and on anterior guidance.

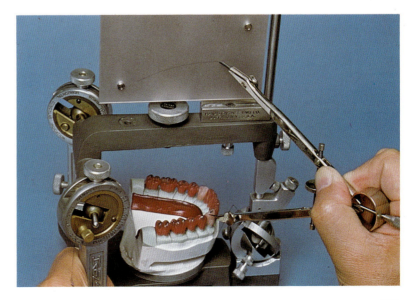

An arch with a radius of 4 inches is drawn on the plastic sheet attached to the flag.

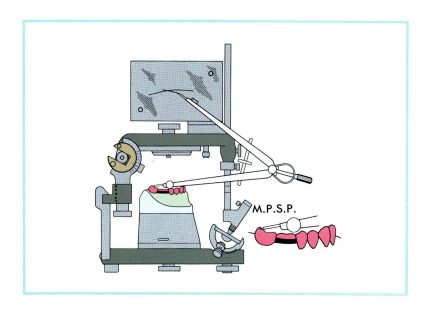

The M.P.S.P. (molar posterior survey point) is placed on the disto-buccal cusp tip of the mandibular second molar. A 4-inch radius arch is scribed on the flag. This is intersected with the A.S.P. line (illustration courtesy of the P.M.S. Manual).

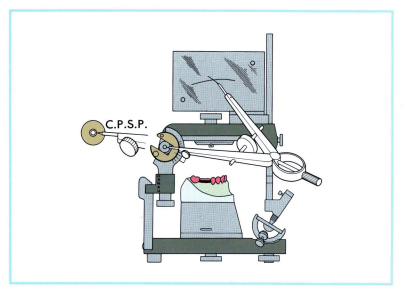

The C.P.S.P. (condylar posterior survey point) is placed on the anterior side of the condylar shaft to scribe a curve, as seen in the illustration above (illustration courtesy of the P.M.S. Manual).

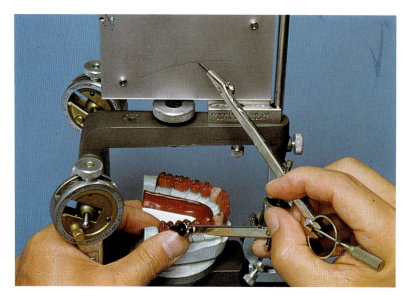

The compass is placed onto the disto-buccal cusp tip of the mandibular second molar and a similar curve is scribed onto the flag (molar posterior survey line).

In some cases, the C.P.S.P. (condylar posterior survey point) is substituted for the M.P.S.P. on the condylar shaft of the articulator, scribing an arch with a diameter of 4 inches.

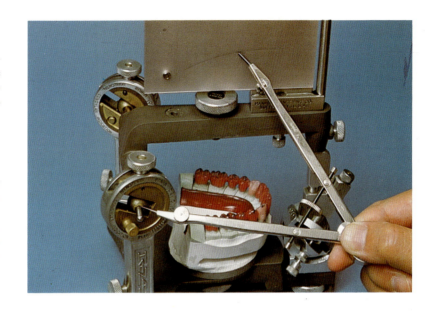

The point at which either the M.P.S.P. or the C.P.S.P. crosses with the A.S.P. arch (A.S.P. line) is determined. From this point, a landmark, O.P.S.C. (occlusal plane survey center), is postulated on the A.S.P. line. Thus the occlusal plane, as indicated by the curve of the Spee, can be established later in the process.

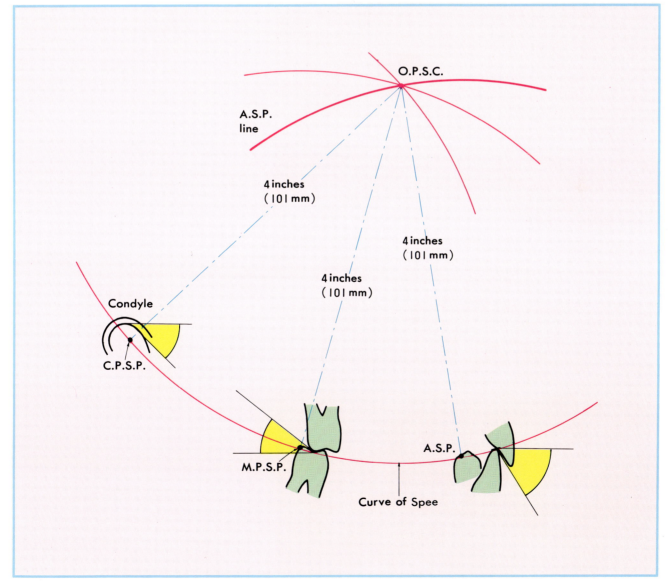

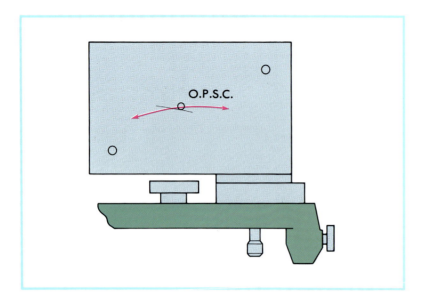

When the central point of the O.P.S.C., used to draw an arch on the mandibular cusps, is placed before the bisecting point on the A.S.P. line, the cusps of the mandibular molars tend to become higher. On the other hand, when the central point is placed posteriorly to the bisecting point, the cusps become lower. This principle deserves our attention. In practice, the bisecting point is determined by placing one end of the compass on the A.S.P. line, thus determining its relationship to the opposing teeth and also finding the degree of the anterior guidances. One method to obtain the O.P.S.C. on the A.S.P. line is shown here (illustration courtesy of the P.M.S. Manual).

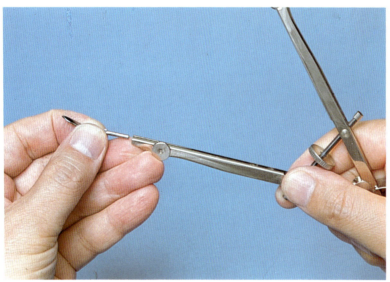

Here the carbon tip of the compass is exchanged with a cutting knife.

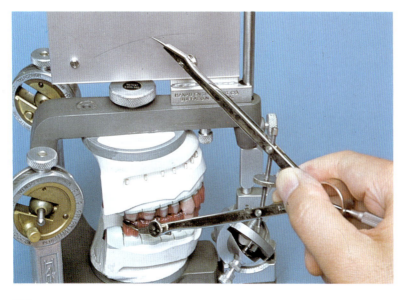

In this stage, the maxillary model is mounted on the articulator and the O.P.S.C. is established on the A.S.P. line by checking the distance between the maxillary and mandibular abutments and the thickness of the material used. As a working guide, the cutting knife should fit between the maxillary and mandibular abutments.

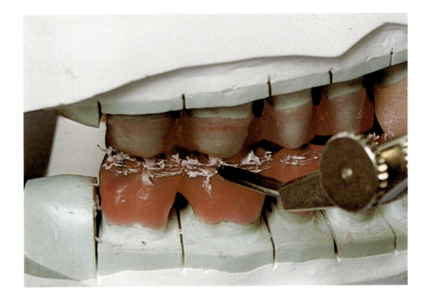

A knife is placed between the maxillary and mandibular abutments. When the O.P.S.C. is thus determined, the upper model can be removed.

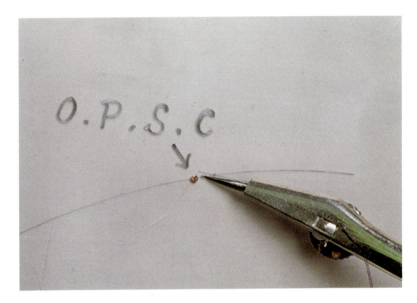

The O.P.S.C. is set somewhat posterior to the bisecting point on the A.S.P. line. A hole is drilled on the O.P.S.C. for the retention of the compass and, in a similar manner, the O.P.S.C. is established on the opposite side.

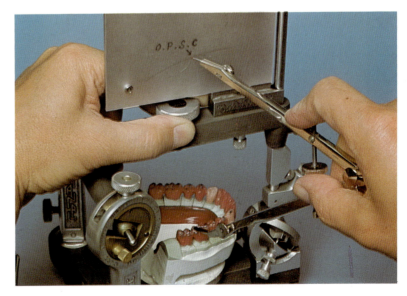

By heating the carving knife, the mandibular occlusal portion is carved by drawing an arch with the compass held firmly on the O.P.S.C.

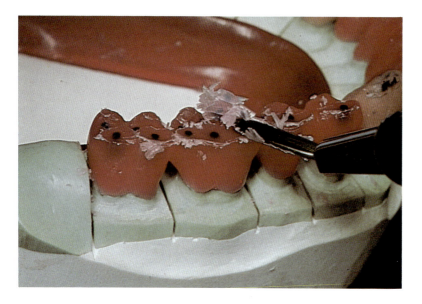

The occlusal surface of the right posterior region is completed by carving the previously established occlusal plane, as originally planned. Thus, the curve of Spee is obtained. The curve of Wilson remains unaffected. This carving procedure should be performed carefully, removing small increments and narrowing the radius of the compass gradually to produce the final 4-inch radius.

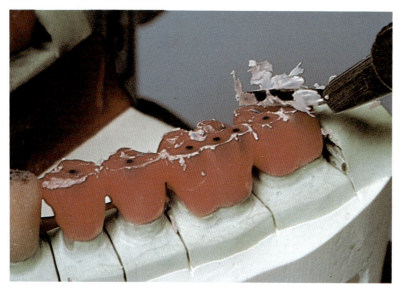

The occlusal plane on the opposite side is treated in a similar manner. Since the wax rods are implanted into the occlusal points, the necessary landmarks are clearly visible.

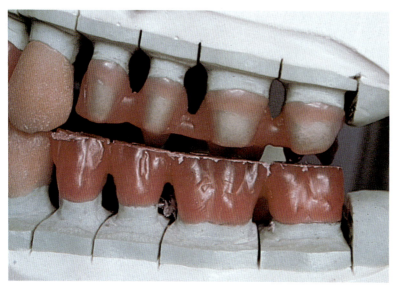

Buccal view of the occlusal surfaces of the left molars.

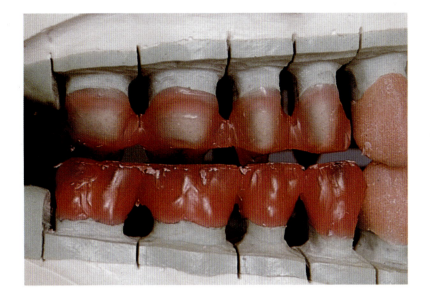

Buccal view of the occlusal plane of the right molars.

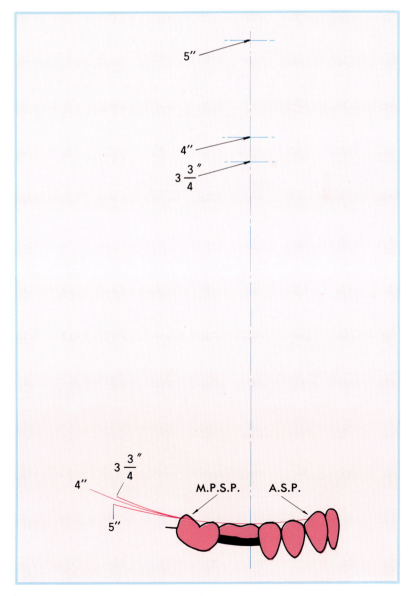

When establishing the occlusal plane, the degree of curvature becomes abrupt if it is more than 4-inches in diameter. This fact should be kept in mind when the occlusal plane is established. As Monson states, a radius of 4 inches is appropriate for almost all cases (illustration: Courtesy P.M.S. Manual).

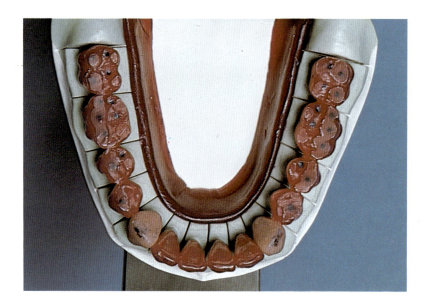

After the mandibular occlusal plane has been established, our next step will be the completion of the molars, based on informaton gained during preceding procedures.

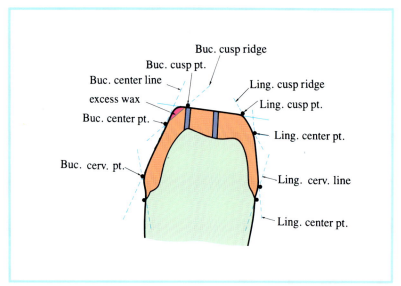

Buc. cusp ridge

Buc. cusp pt.

Buc. center line

Ling. cusp ridge

excess wax

Ling. cusp pt.

Buc. center pt.

Ling. center pt.

Buc. cerv. pt.

Ling. cerv. line

Ling. center pt.

The buccal cusp points have been determined, and in the next step, excess wax is cut off from the buccal surface and buccal cusp tips in order to create the buccal cusp line. The lingual cusp tip is now waxed up. Remember that the distance between the cusps accounts for 55 to 60% of the crown length. Thus, an outline, relating to the three previously discussed planes, is obtained.

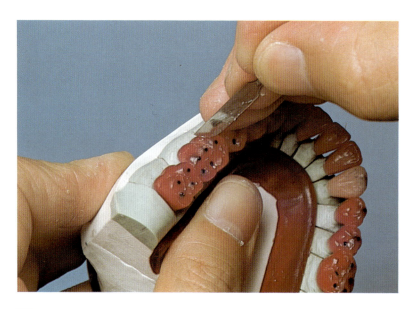

On the mandibular first molar, the buccal cuspal plane extends from the buccal center line to the buccal cusp tips.

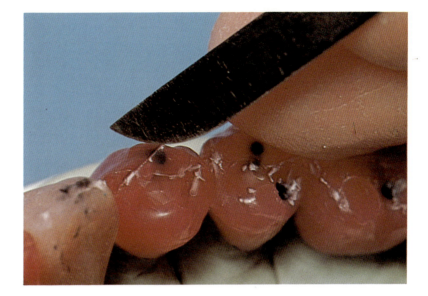

After completion of the mesial buccal cuspal plane, the same process is continued for the center part and for the distal aspects of the first premolars.

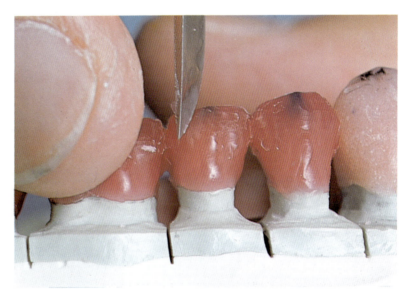

The buccal cusp plane for the second premolar is formed in a similar manner.

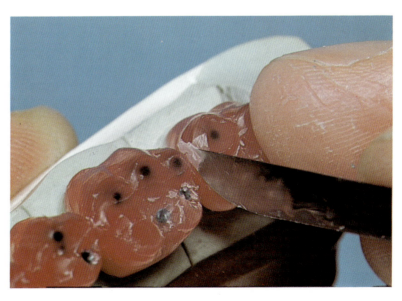

After completion of the buccal cusp plane, contour adjustments are necessary.

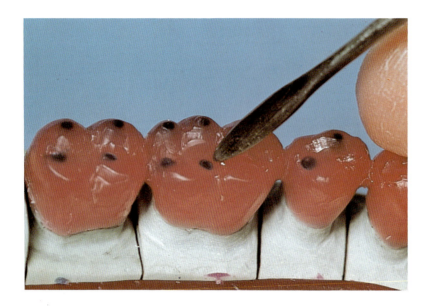

The formation of the buccal and lingual cusp planes provides the angle of disengagement. If it appears that this angle should be greater, a small amount of wax can be added near the central fossa. The color coding of waxes guarantees the distinction of the later addition of wax from the wax rods.

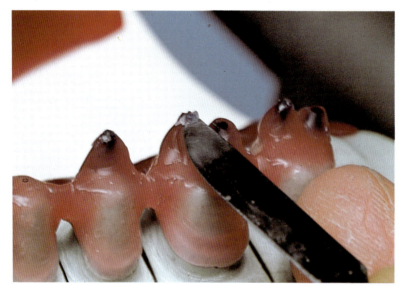

When wax is added in the central fossae, it is advantageous to shorten the tips of the lingual cusps of the opposing teeth. If we want to design the freedom from C.R.O. on the lower molar, we will transfer the wax pattern into acrylic resin.

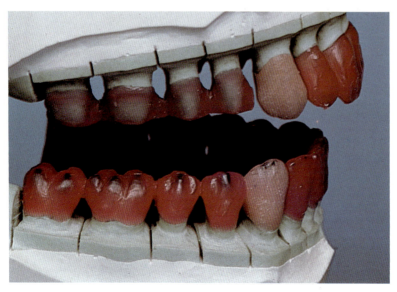

A buccal view of the right mandibular molar region with all procedures completed.

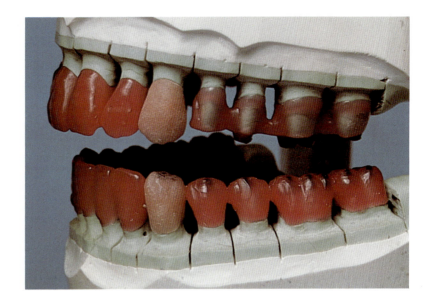

A lateral view of the left posterior region.

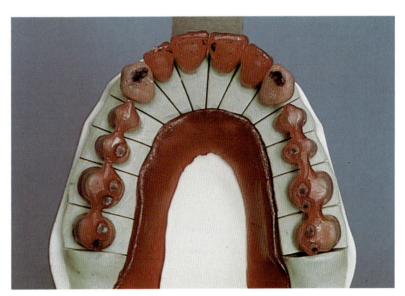

An occlusal view of the maxillary arch.

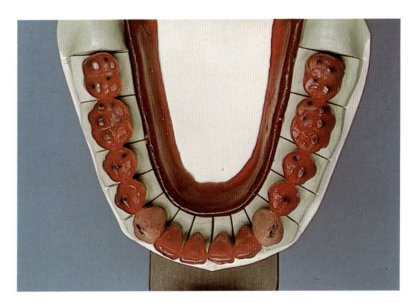

An occlusal view of the mandibular arch. The only remaining procedural step is the establishment of the angle of disengagement.

3.3.7. DISENGAGEMENT OF MOLAR CUSPS; ESTABLISHING INCLINED PLANE

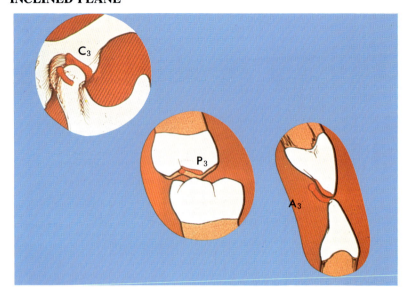

In a protrusive movement of the mandible, the respective molar cusps should not be in occlusal contact with the opposing teeth; the degree of this disocclusion is dependent on the degree of anterior guidance and condylar inclination. (illustration: Dr. P. Neff: Occlusion and Function)

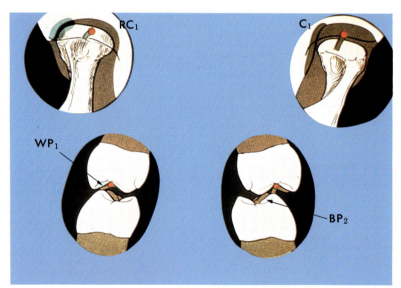

In lateral mandibular movement, the respective molar cusps on the balancing side should not come into occlusal contact with the opposing teeth. Here again, the degree of disocclusion is determined by the degree of anterior guidance, the Bennet movement, and the condylar movement on the balancing side. (illustration: Dr. P. Neff: Occlusion and Function)

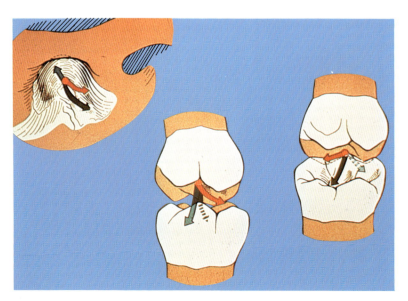

The mandibular movement and the functional anatomy of the teeth are illustrated two-dimensionally: they must be **imagined** as a three-dimensional pattern. This fact should be always kept in mind. (illustration courtesy from Dr. P. Neff: Occlusion and Function)

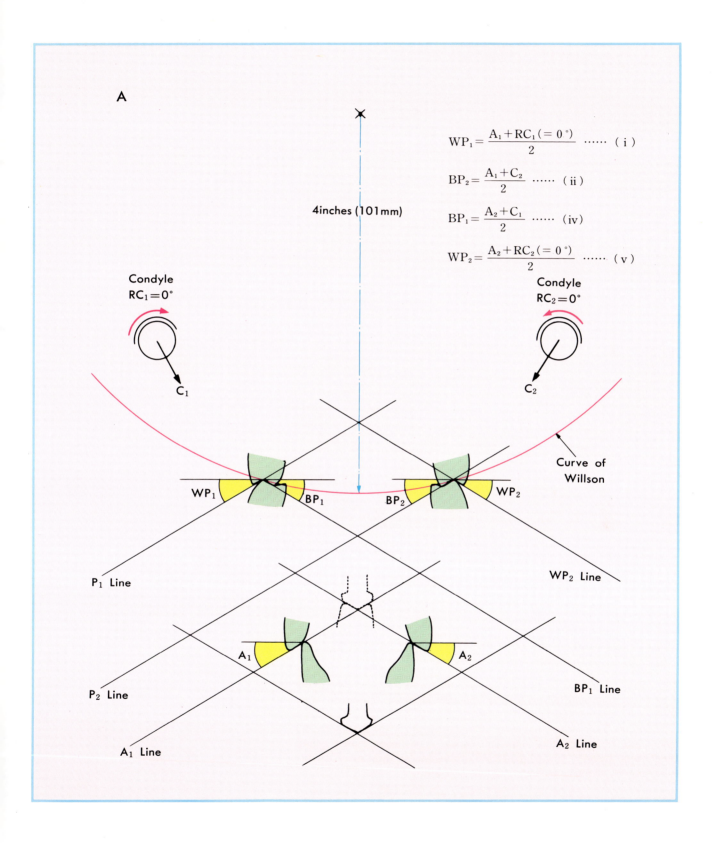

A

$$WP_1 = \frac{A_1 + RC_1 (= 0°)}{2} \quad \cdots\cdots \; (\,i\,)$$

$$BP_2 = \frac{A_1 + C_2}{2} \quad \cdots\cdots \; (\,ii\,)$$

$$BP_1 = \frac{A_2 + C_1}{2} \quad \cdots\cdots \; (\,iv\,)$$

$$WP_2 = \frac{A_2 + RC_2 (= 0°)}{2} \quad \cdots\cdots \; (\,v\,)$$

4 inches (101 mm)

Condyle
$RC_1 = 0°$

C_1

Condyle
$RC_2 = 0°$

C_2

Curve of
Willson

WP_1 BP_1 BP_2 WP_2

P_1 Line

WP_2 Line

P_2 Line

A_1 A_2

BP_1 Line

A_1 Line

A_2 Line

Determination of deployment angles for the mandibular molars in lateral movement.

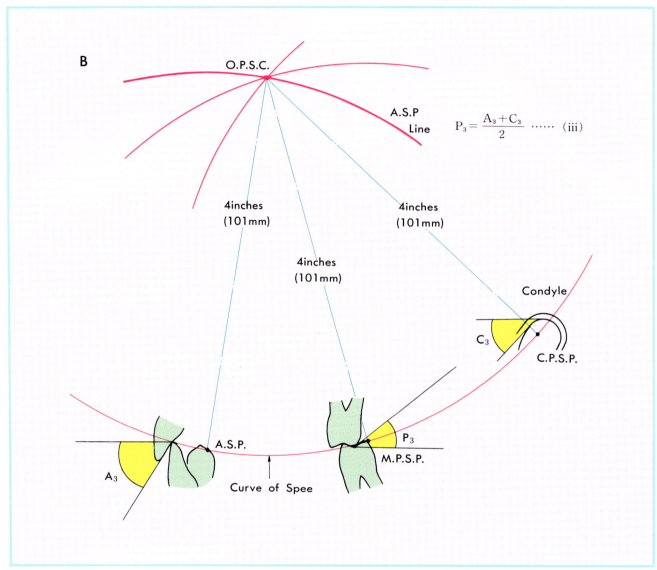

B

O.P.S.C.

A.S.P Line

$$P_3 = \frac{A_3 + C_3}{2} \quad \cdots\cdots \quad (iii)$$

4inches (101mm)

4inches (101mm)

4inches (101mm)

Condyle

C_3

C.P.S.P.

A.S.P.

P_3

M.P.S.P.

A_3

Curve of Spee

Determination of deployment angles for the mandibular molars in forward movement.

A. DETERMINATION OF DEPLOYMENT ANGLES FOR THE MANDIBULAR MOLARS

The condylar angles C_1 and C_2 are set on the articulator. When the mandibular right and left canines are engaged in lateral movement, they move in the direction of angles A_1 and A_2.

When providing proper angles of disengagement for the maxillary and mandibular teeth, we must know the mode of occlusion: either **group function occluson** or **canine protected occlusion**. For this procedure, the following set of mathematical equations is helpful.

1) The inclination angle BP_1 for the molars on the balancing side during the left lateral movement.

$$BP_1 = \frac{A_2 + C_1}{2} \cdot \cdot \cdot \cdot \cdot (iv)$$

where,
A_2 = The anterior guidance angle on the working side during the left lateral movement
C_1 = The condylar path on the balancing side

2) The inclination angle WP_2 for molars on the working side during left lateral movement.

$$WP_2 = \frac{A_2 + RC_2(=0°)}{2} \quad \ldots \ldots \text{(v)}$$

where

A_2 = The angle on the working side during the left lateral anterior guidance movement

RC_2 = The condyle rotation on the working side ($RC_2 = 0°$)

The lingual cuspal inclination of the mandibular molars on the working side must be reduced from whatever angle is parallel to the WP_2 line.

From the equations above, we can obtain approximate figures of deployment angles. It follows: $180° - (WP_1 + BP_1)$ or $180° - (BP_2 + WP_2)$. However, it is clinically impractical to use these numerical values.

As a practical alternative, we can move the articulator in all excursions with reference to the anterior guidance. With this simple method, approximate values are dynamically obtained.

As described by P.E. Dawson (Dawson 1974), the surface of the incisal table on the articulator is filled in with wax, and after moving the pin laterally to the right and left, the approximate angle of disengagement can be registered (based on the anterior guidance of the resin canine) with the incisal pin on the wax. By embedding some epoxy resin into the wax, we can obtain an exact record of the disengagement angle for any given patient.

B. PROVISION OF DISENGAGEMENT ANGLES FOR THE MANDIBULAR MOLAR INCLINES ON THE SAGITTAL PLANE

The inclination P_3 for the mandibular molar cusps, as viewed sagittally, is expressed in the following equation.

$$P_3 = \frac{A_3 + C_3}{2} \quad \ldots \ldots \text{(iii)}$$

where

A_3 = Anterior guidance angle during the forward movement

C_3 = Condylar path on the sagittal plane

With forward movement, the resultant numerical value must be decreased (below the number derived from the equation) to avoid occlusal contact between molars.

In other words, when the incisal overbite is shallow and the sagittal condylar path is similarly shallow, the value of P_3 needs to remain correspondingly shallow. If it is too deep, molar interference in the forward movement is the result.

When establishing angles for the cuspal inclinations of the mandibular molars on the sagittal plane, the degree of anterior overbite and the condylar angles must be examined carefully.

In order to create a disocclusion in a protrusive movement in the molar region, the sagittal condylar angle needs to be properly adjusted on the articulator.

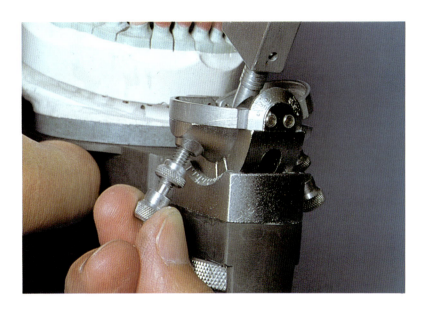

Beginning with this illustration, a series of procedural steps for the establishment of disengagement angles is shown. In order to start with the anterior guidance table, the Hanau articulator (Model 145-2) is adjusted to 0°.

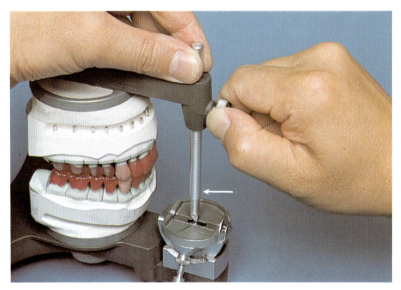

The adjustable incisal pin is removed and replaced with the Hanau cusp fossa pin (see arrow). Even if this adjustable incisal pin is removed, the vertical dimension is stablized through the resin canines.

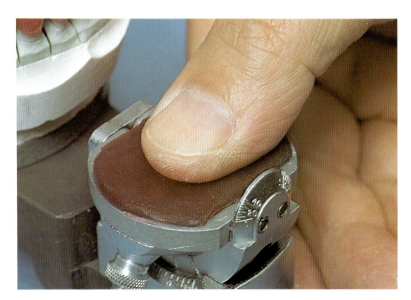

The surface of the anterior guidance table is filled in with wax.

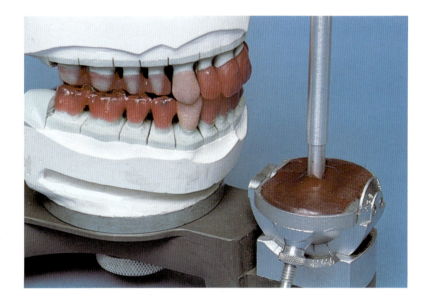

The incisal pin is inserted into the wax on the anterior guidance table.

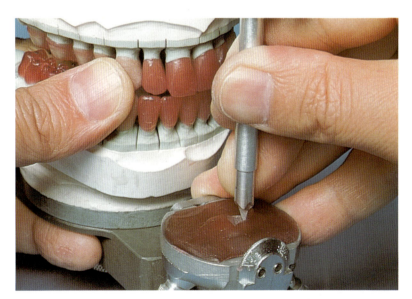

The articulator is moved laterally. The anterior guidance of the resin canine serves as a reference.

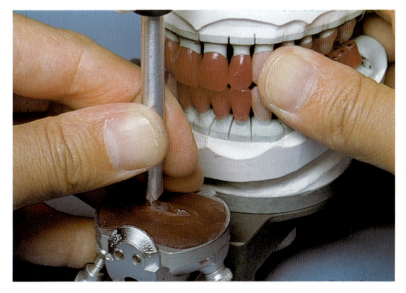

In the lateral movement, we check for the presence of contact. Since the wax offers some resistance, we have to compensate for this when moving the pin. This step shows lateral movement to the left side.

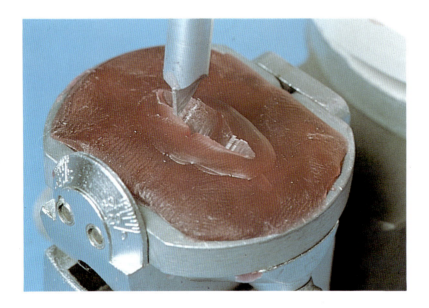

The guide for the disengagement angle of the mandibular molars as registered in wax with the incisal pin.

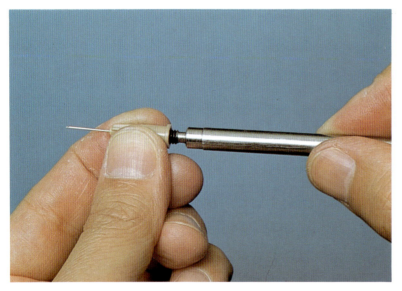

The incisal pin is removed from the articulator. An injection needle is inserted in the tip of the extension pin.

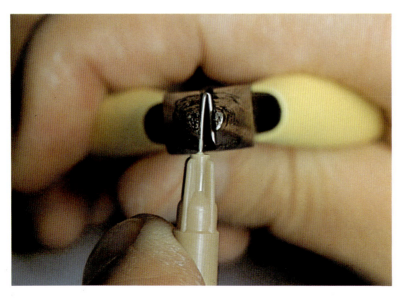

The tip of the needle is bent to facilitate retention.

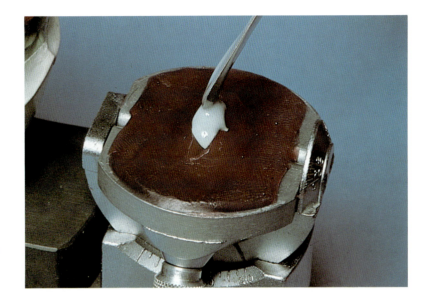

In order to produce a lock model, a small amount of epoxy resin is filled into the concavity previously created with the incisal pin.

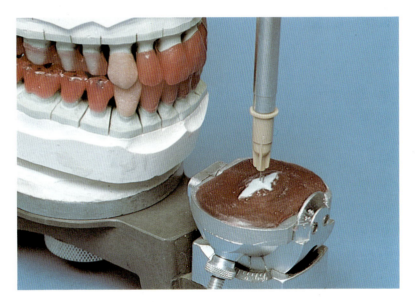

During the next step, the bent extension pin is inserted into the resin before it sets completely.

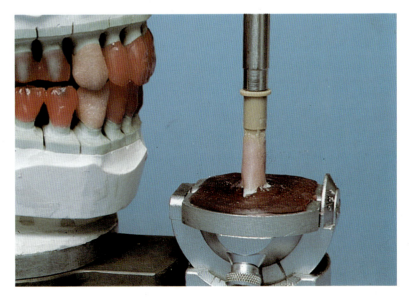

After the lock model has been completely set, it and the needle portion are joined together with self-curing acrylic resin.

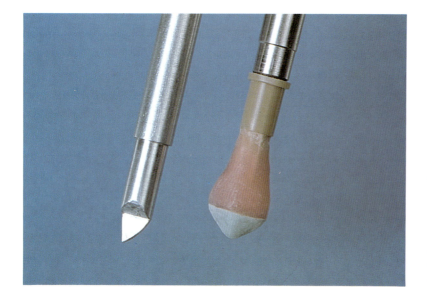

Left: The cusp fossa pin used for the procedure illustrated above.

Right: The finished custom-made cusp fossa instrument.

The angles of disengagement obtained with such an instrument have their application in the molar region. The actual determination of the disengagement angles is influenced by A_1 and A_2 (as obtained from the anterior guidance), and for this reason, information concerning the C_1 and C_2 is relatively sparse.

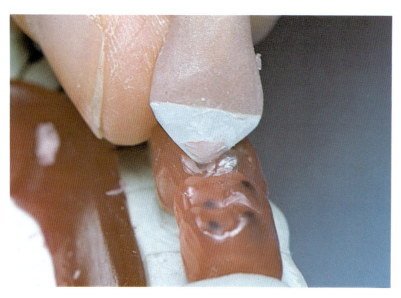

Note:
1) The anterior guidance being shallow, it is difficult to execute the angle of disengagement deeply enough.
2) With a shallow condylar path, it is difficult to execute the angle of disengagement with sufficient depth.
3) The angle of disengagement becomes shallower as the molar region is approached.

The last consideration is necessary in order to avoid a possible cuspal interference in the molar region. If this occurred, the temporomandibular joint would be adversely affected. The more distal the cuspal interference encountered, the more severe the adverse affect.

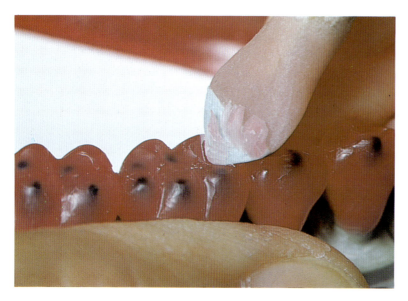

The tip of the instrument is placed into the central fossa, and by using its flat part, the wax is carved to provide the correct angle of disengagement.

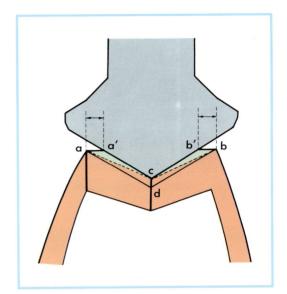

In order to reduce the angle of disengagement as we go toward the last molar, the procedure illustrated here is followed.

1. Since the occlusal plane is already determined through the Broadlick occlusal plane analyzer, points **a** and **b** should not be touched during the procedure.
2. The respective area between a–a' and b–b' must be smooth and uniform. Thus it will be possible to render the angle of disengagement as shallow as necessary by moving the tip of the instrument from **d** to **c.**
3. A shallow angle of disengagement will produce the form of △a'cb' and, is created by cutting △aca' and △bcb'.

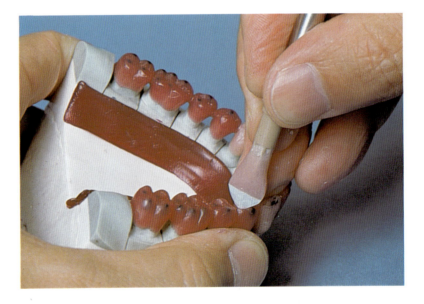

When the disengagement angle of the mandibular molars is carved too deep, it is impossible to achieve contact between the maxillary molar cusp ridges and the mandibular central fossae. Yet if it is too shallow, masticatory efficiency is reduced. Therefore, when establishing the angle of disengagement, major consideration must be given to harmony between anterior guidance and the condylar angle. Therefore, both angles (anterior and posterior guidances) must be shallower than the inclination angles of the molar cusps.

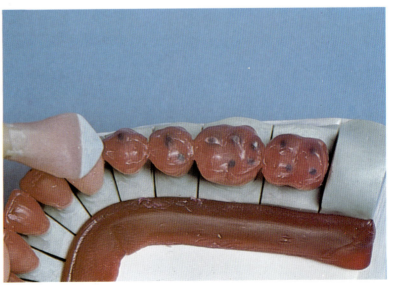

In the procedures illustrated above, we have established the following:

1. Functional crown contour
2. Occlusal plane
3. Disengagement angle (cusp-fossa relationship)
4. The cuspal inclination angles as viewed from the sagittal plane.

On the planning wax crown, grooves and minor ridges are not established. Next, the functional guidance is manufactured as an index of the occlusal surfaces of the mandibular molars, and used as a guide for building up the porcelain on the occlusal surface. When preparing a complete cast crown, grooves and even minor ridges are registered on the diagnostic wax-up.

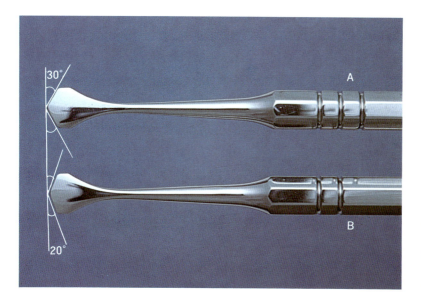

This illustration shows two stock cusp fossa instruments of different angulation.

A shows a 100° angulation with 30° cusp fossa angulation.

B shows a 140° angulation with 20° cusp fossa angulation.

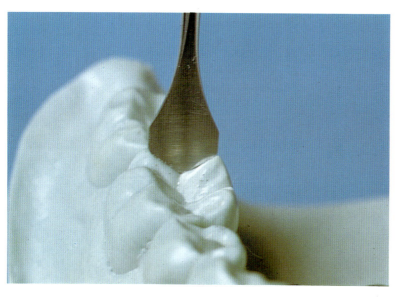

The correctly angulated instrument is selected and its use demonstrated on the cast.

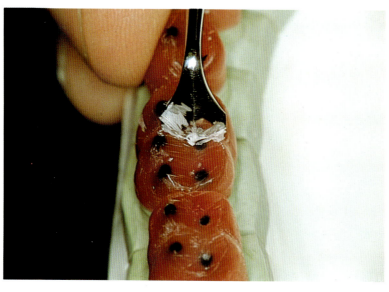

Correct application of the instrument on the planning crown for the first molar. Following establishment of cusp fossa angulation on the planning wax-up, the wax-up procedure is completed **without** forming any grooves.

3.3.8. DESIGN OF THE MOLAR WAX CROWN (SKELETAL TECHNIQUE)

The planning wax-up for a large ceramometal restoration has already been discussed. When teeth remain on the side opposite the restoration, it is much easier to obtain necessary landmark points to serve as an overall frame of reference.

In the following illustrations, a maxillary first molar is used to demonstrate the fabrication of a full cast crown utilizing the skeletal technique and the three dimensional waxing technique.

In the presence of the adjacent teeth and the teeth on the opposite side of the arch, the wax patterns must be constructed following the sequence listed below.

① Mesiobuccal cusp point
② Distobuccal cusp point
③ Distal cusp point
④ Central occlusal point
⑤ (Distal) central occlusal point
⑥ Lingual (mesial) cuspal point
⑦ Lingual (distal) cuspal point
⑧ Buccal mesial point
⑨ Buccal distal point
⑩ (mesial) marginal ridge point
⑪ (distal) marginal ridge point
⑫ Buccal (mesial) cervical point
⑬ Buccal (distal) cervical point
⑭ Lingual cervical point (mesial)
⑮ Lingual cervical point (distal)
⑯ Lingual mesial point
⑰ Lingual distal point

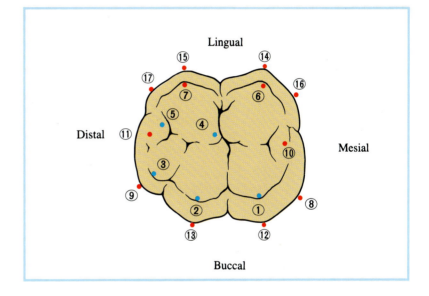

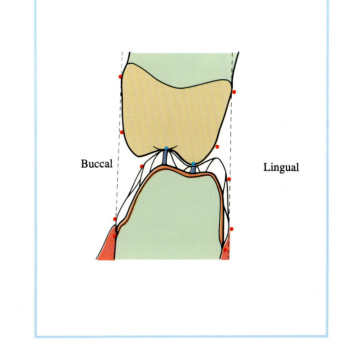

Here, the wax rods are implanted on the lingual cusp tips in the direction of the maxillary lingual cusp tips. The basic skeletons are built up by joining the involved structures with wax and subsequently waxing them up completely, following the three plane concept.

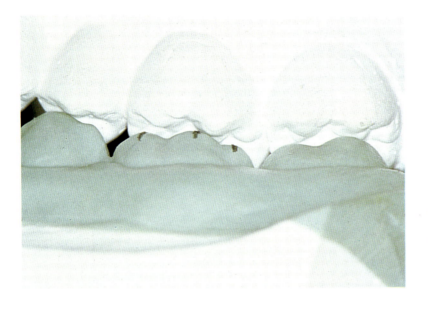

The respective positions of the buccal cusp ridges for the teeth on the opposite side are marked in order to find the distances between the buccal cusp ridges and their corresponding occlusal contacts on the opposing teeth. These are used simply for reference, not as guides per se.

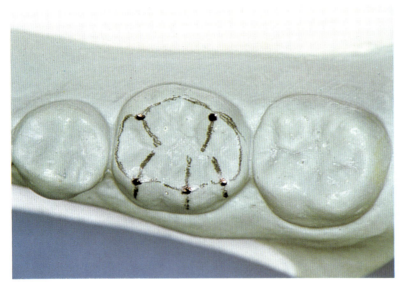

The occlusal view of the marked grooves and secondary ridges serves as reference.

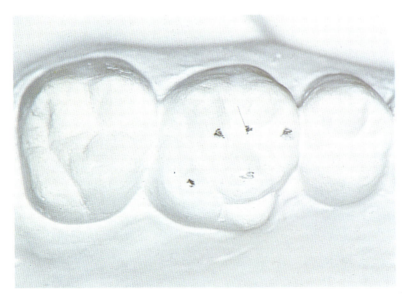

The lingual cusp tips are marked by the opposing teeth and the occlusal surface of the restoration in its final form is planned now.

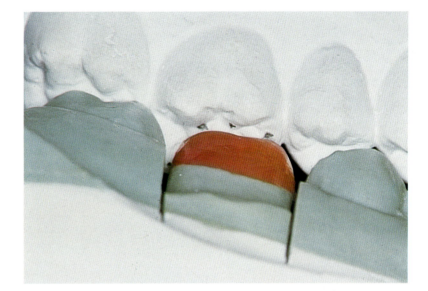

The sheet wax coping of the mandibular arch is brought into C.O. contact with the maxillary arch and the wax rod is luted to the coping.

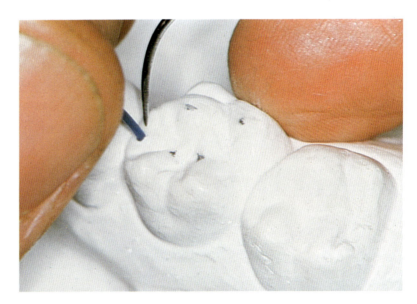

Subsequently, the mandible is moved and its functional relationship with the maxillary arch confirmed.

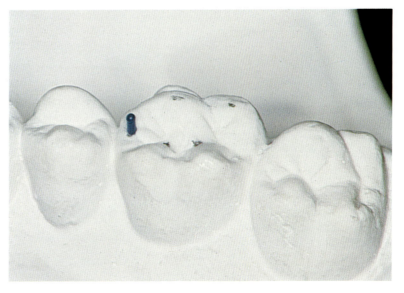

Here the buccal cuspal point is obtained for the mandibular first molar.

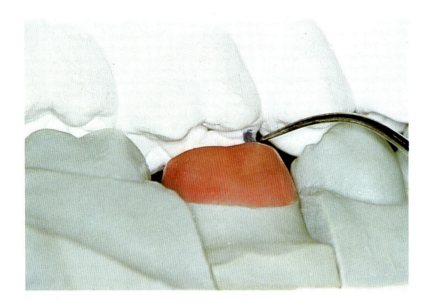

After positioning the wax rod on the mesial marginal ridge of the wax first molar, the casts are brought into occlusion. Upon opening, we find the wax rod luted to the mesiobuccal cusp tip point ① of the coping of the mandibular first molar.

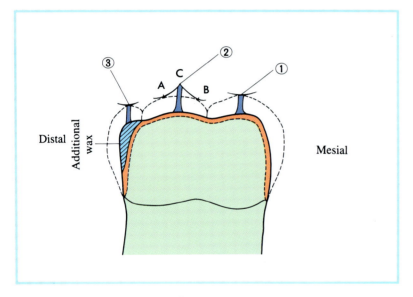

Similarly, the wax rod is placed on the distal buccal cusp tip. If the disto-buccal cusp tip does not come into occlusal contact, the wax rod is implanted in the central groove (indicated by C), because the main purpose of the placement is to establish an adequate occlusal relationship between the maxillary and mandibular arches.

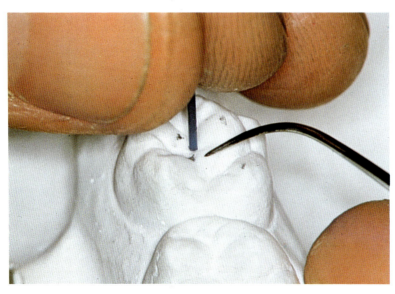

A wax rod is placed on the central fossa (C as indicated above).

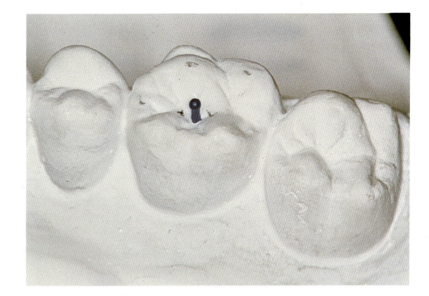

A wax rod is implanted on the central fossa, and its length properly determined. Thus the buccal occlusal point is established, ②.

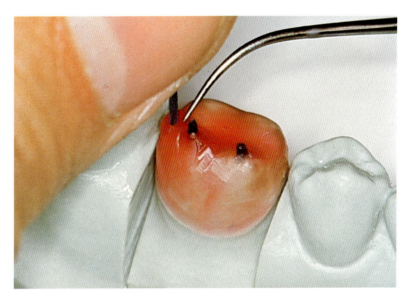

The respective wax rods, ② and ③, are joined with the coping. Now a check is made for cuspal interferences between the wax rods and cusps of the opposing teeth. The absence of cuspal interference is confirmed through mandibular movement, ③.

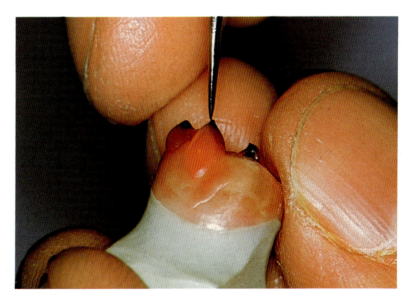

After the wax rods have been placed on the respective buccal cusps, their bases are reinforced with wax. This results in a cone-shaped appearance.

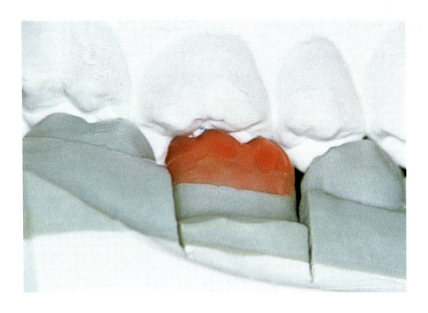

After the reinforcement of the wax rods, the occlusal contacts are roughly determined for a final occlusion check.

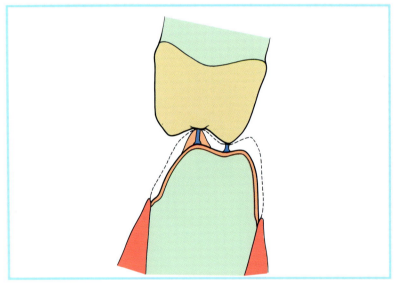

The wax rods are placed on the mesial and distal lingual cusp tips of the opposing tooth and are luted to the coping.

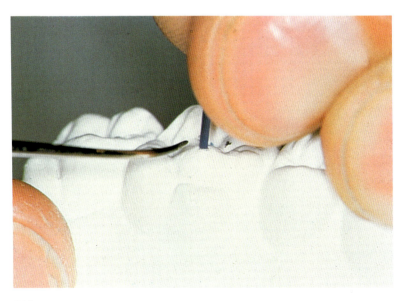

The wax rods are placed on the mesiolingual cusp tip of the opposing tooth, parallel to its long axis.

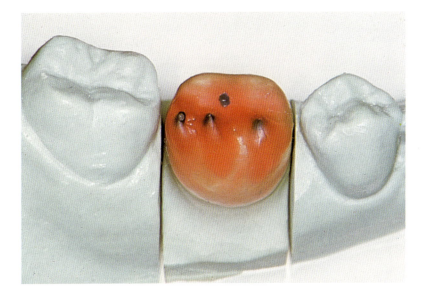

The wax rods placed on the mesio-lingual cusp tips of the opposing teeth are joined with the copings, ④.

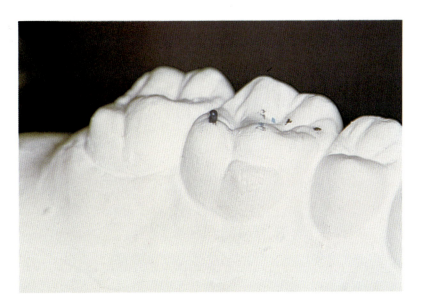

The wax rods are placed on the disto-lingual cusp tip of the opposing tooth.

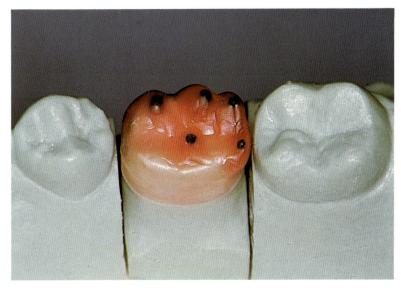

The central fossa point is established by joining the wax rod on the disto-lingual cusp tip with the copings. Except for the wax rod directed to the central fossa of the maxillary molar, all the rods come into occlusal contact with their opposing teeth. Now they are positioned correctly, (① − ⑤).

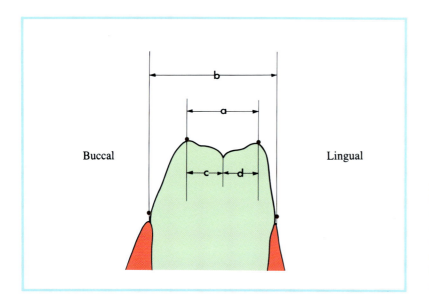

The distance between the buccal and lingual cusps **A** accounts for about 55 to 60% of the buccolingual maximum width of the crown **B**; the distance between the buccal cusp tip and the central fossa **C** is almost equal to the distance between the lingual cusp tips and the central fossae **D**. These values help us plan construction of the final crown contour.

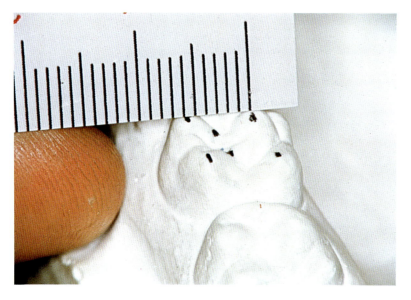

The above distances, **A, B,** and **C** are measured on the opposing teeth. From this, we learn that $\mathbf{A} = \mathbf{B} \times (0.55 \sim 0.60)$, $\mathbf{C} = \mathbf{D}$.

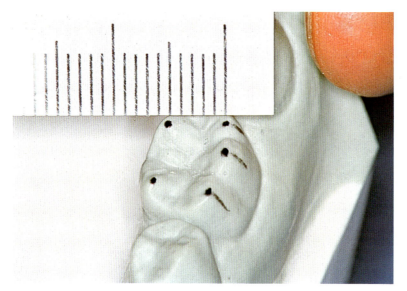

The same distances are measured on the teeth of the opposite side. In this particular case, the values approximate those of the opposing teeth.

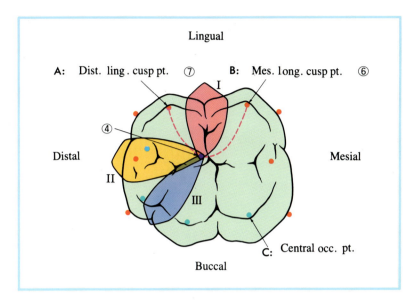

Now the mesial and distal cusps are waxed up. In this instance, an equilateral triangle is formed by the mesial and distal lingual cusp tips and the tip of the wax rod is placed in the central fossa, the red dotted line indicating the ridge leading to the central fossa. Of the three directions of movement from I to III, the distance between the mesial and distal lingual cusps is the largest (A–B); therefore, interference of the maxillary mesial lingual cusps must be avoided during movement on the working side.

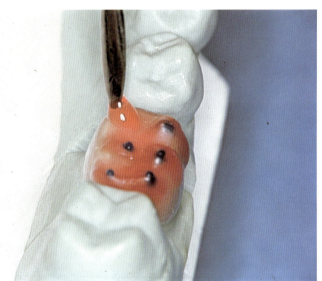

With consideration of the above, the position of the mesial lingual cusps is determined. They are then built up conically, ⑥.

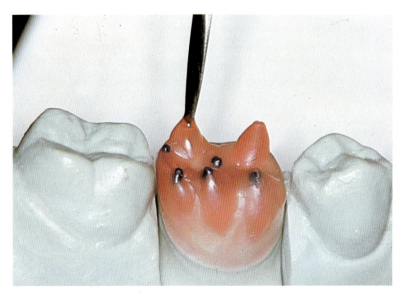

The disto-lingual cusp is similarly prepared in conical form, ⑦.

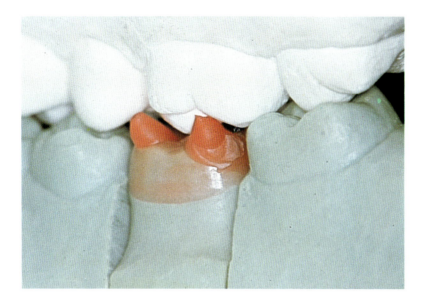

The disto-lingual cusp tips are directed toward the distal lingual grooves of the opposing teeth.

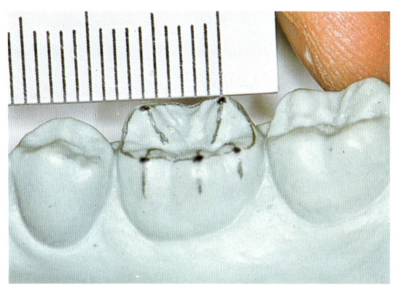

The distances between the same teeth of the opposite side provide the criteria for formation of the mesial and distal lingual cusps of the restorations.

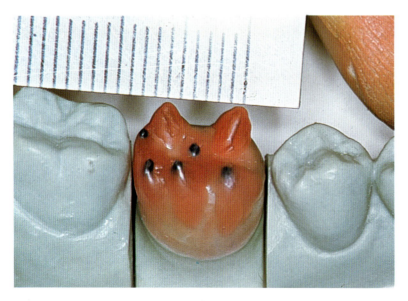

The distance between the prepared mesial and disto-lingual cusps is confirmed by measurement.

The buccal mesial point largely influences the contour of the maxillary buccal surfaces, ⑧.

Attention must be paid to their functional relationship with the adjacent teeth and associated tissues.

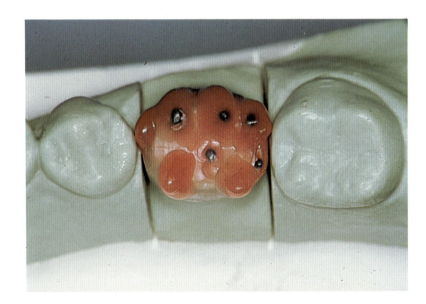

The buccal distal point is waxed up in relation to the second molar, keeping in mind the morphological and functional aspects of the teeth, ⑨.

Occlusal view after completion of the wax-up.

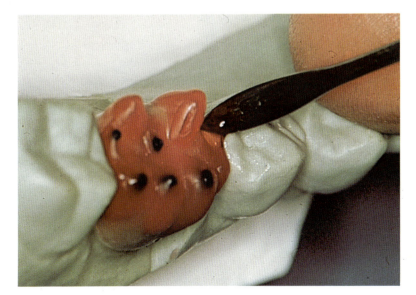

With due considerations of the adjacent teeth, the mesial marginal ridge point is constructed, ⑩ and ⑪.

In the next step, the distal marginal ridge point is waxed up.

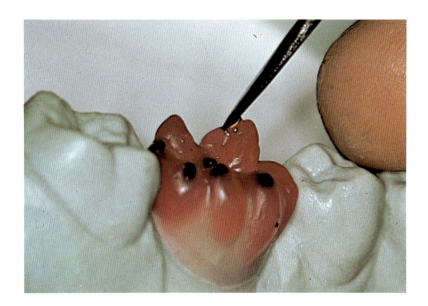

The ridges leading to the lingual groove are supplemented with wax in order to reproduce the natural contour, ⑥.

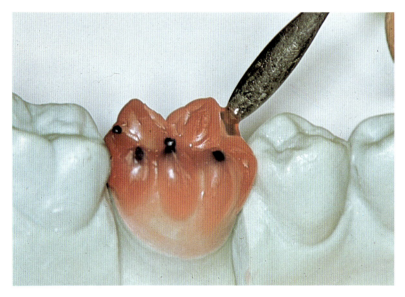

The lingual cuspal points and marginal ridges are joined in order to complete the contour of the lingual ridges, ⑥ and ⑩.

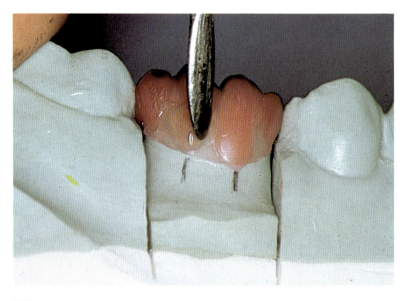

The buccal cusp ridges are waxed up. The highest point of the cusp ridges close to the cervix will constitute the height of contour, ⑫ and ⑬.

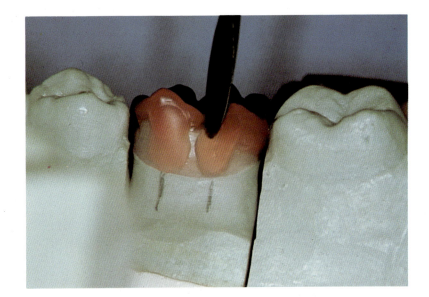

The lingual cusp ridges are waxed up, ⑭ and ⑮.

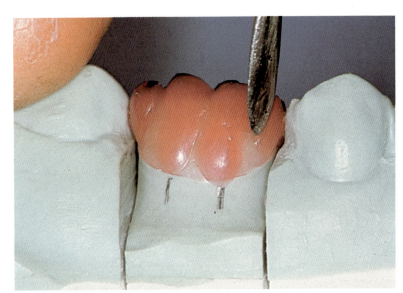

The areas between the buccal cusp ridges are filled in with wax, ⑯ and ⑰.

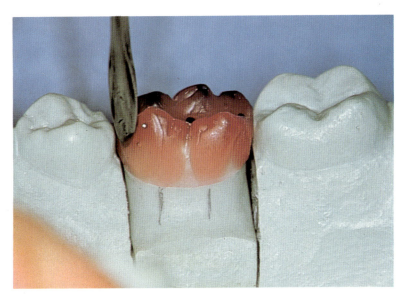

The mesial and distal cusp ridges on the lingual surface are filled in with wax, ⑧ and ⑨.

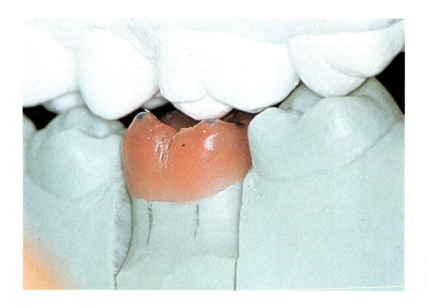

Up to this stage, the crown contour of the mandibular right first molar has been nearly completed. The illustration shows the occlusal contacts on the first molar.

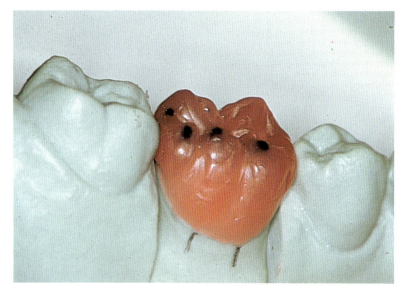

At this time, final crown contour is nearly completed. Only minor modifications remain. An occlusal view of an extracted natural mandibular first molar is shown here. From comparison with the natural tooth, it is evident that the skeletal technique does enable us to create a physiological and anatomically correct restoration.

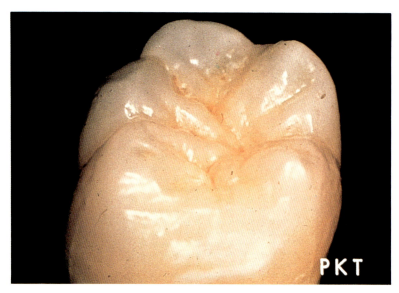

We must be totally familiar with the anatomy of the natural teeth in order to be able to reproduce lost tooth structure. In this sense, nature is the best textbook available (photograph courtesy of Dr. P.K. Thomas).

3.4 ESTABLISHING FUNCTIONAL GUIDANCE

A set of indices is obtained through resin impressions of the occlusal and lateral surfaces of the mandibular planning wax crown. At the same time, the position of the respective cusp tips of the mandibular molars are registered. This set of indices is called a **functional guide.**

By preparing this type of functional guide on the maxillary cast, it is possible to project the entire or partial occlusal surfaces of the mandibular molars in porcelain. The porcelain can be prepared on the indices as initially planned. The functional guide as an index of occlusion for the planning wax-up of the mandibular molars is prepared in the following illustrations. The functional guide can be defined as an occlusal record of the mandibular molars and premolars in a situation in which the occlusal surfaces of the opposing teeth have been either partially or completely lost.

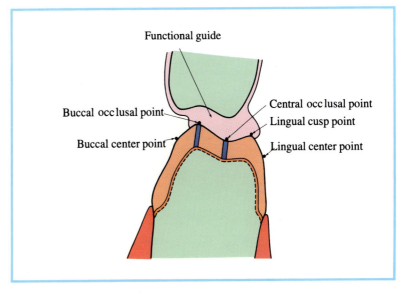

Functional guide

Buccal occlusal point

Central occlusal point

Lingual cusp point

Buccal center point

Lingual center point

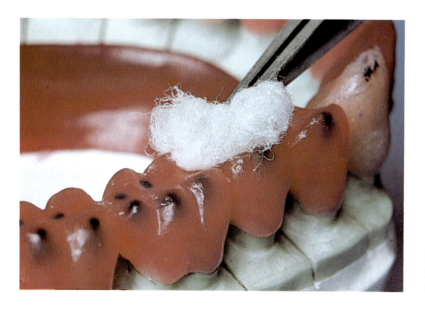

As an initial step in preparing the functional guide, the occlusal surfaces of the mandibular planning wax crowns are coated with vaseline that serves as a separator.

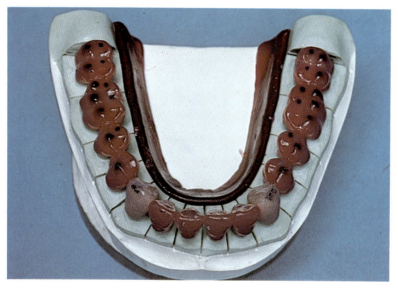

At this time, it may prove useful to take impressions of the molars for future procedures.

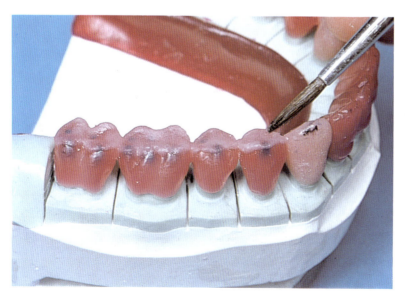

Now the following areas are covered with a thin layer of self-curing resin. They are ① the lingual occlusal points, ② the buccal occlusal points, ③ the marginal ridge points, ④ the central occlusal points, and ⑤ the mesiodistal line angle points.

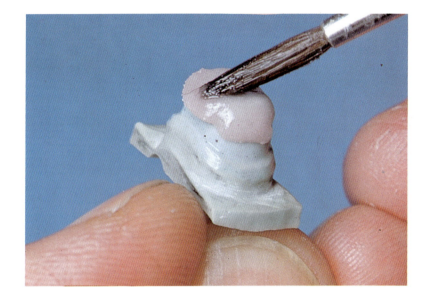

The maxillary molars are also coated with vaseline and their occlusal thirds are covered with the self-curing resin.

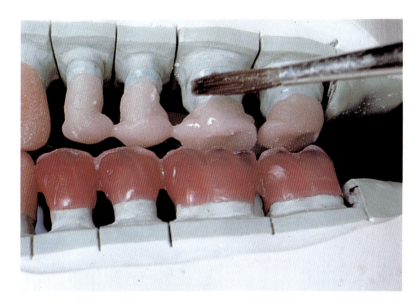

When the resin has set, the copings are cemented at their proximal portions only.

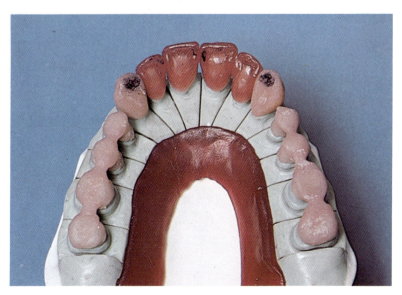

If a defect is detected on the maxillary molars, the defective part is repaired with resin.

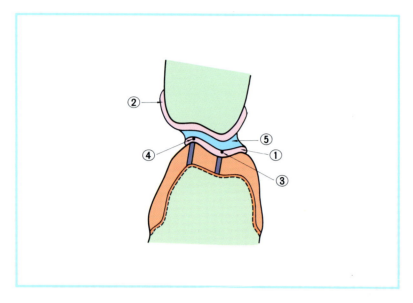

A thin layer of acrylic resin is applied to the occlusal surfaces of the mandibular molars ①. The maxillary molar copings ② must be appropriately spaced; there must be no contact betweem them. In the next step, the central and buccal occlusal points ①, ③, and ④, are marked on the resin and then the maxillary and mandibular resin build-ups, ①, and ②, are joined with resin ⑤.

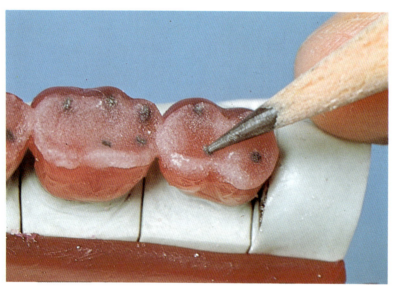

Some resin is also applied to the mandibular occlusal surfaces; the coating must be thin enough to allow the wax rods to show through the resin layer. The necessary points are marked on the resin in pencil.

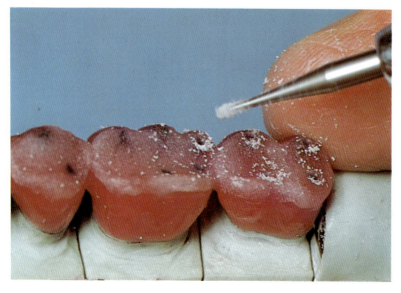

Again, the marked areas are perforated with a bur of a diameter 0.7–0.8mm. The holes should perforate the resin, but not reach the wax pattern.

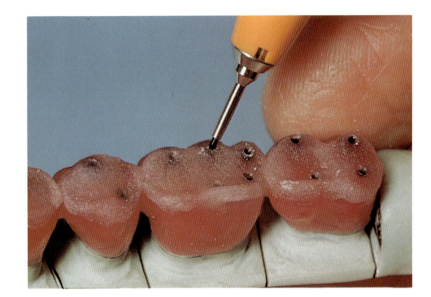

Using a fine waterproof felt pen, the perforated holes are carefully marked.

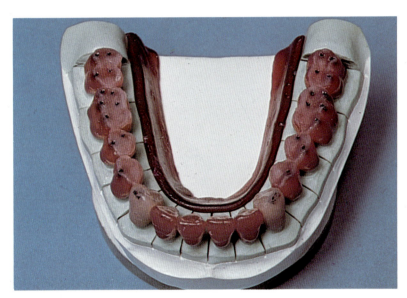

All occlusal surfaces of the mandibular molars have been marked.

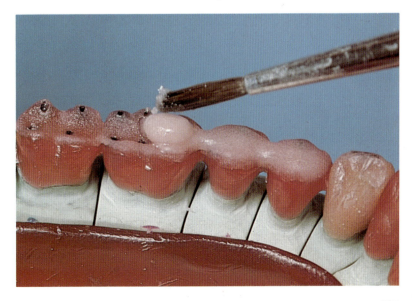

Now more resin is added to the marked resin layer. The amount of resin required is determined by the space between the adjacent teeth. The contacts with the opposing teeth show up as dots.

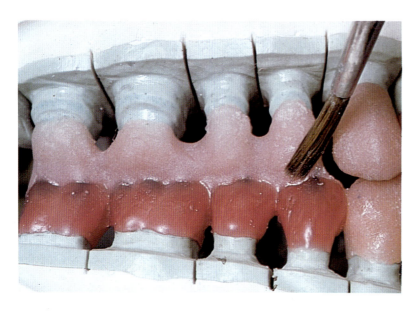

Before the added resin sets up completely, the space between the maxillary and mandibular teeth is filled in with additional resin material. It is absolutely necessary that the maxillary and mandibular resin canines be in correct occlusal contact with each other.

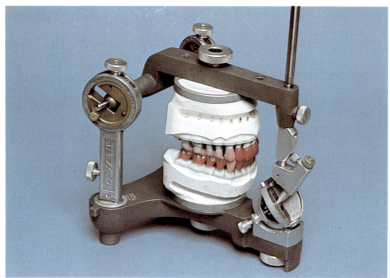

The buccal view of the functional guide; it is imperative that the functional guide have no contact with the resin canines. The resin is allowed to set completely. The fabrication of the functional guide is an important prerequisite for the construction of planning wax crowns for all the mandibular molars.

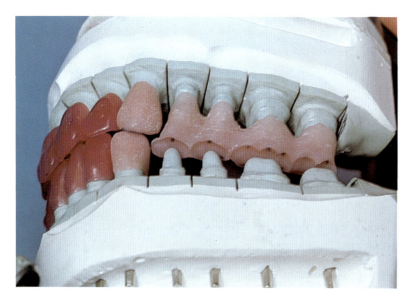

A close up view of the finished functional guide. Notice the occlusal marks: these provide useful guidelines for further operation.

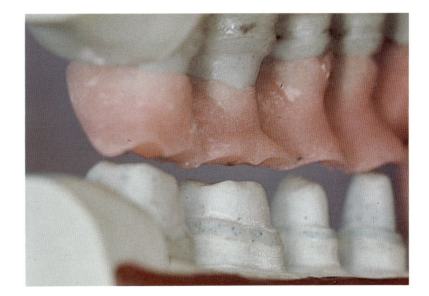

A lingual view of the left functional guide.

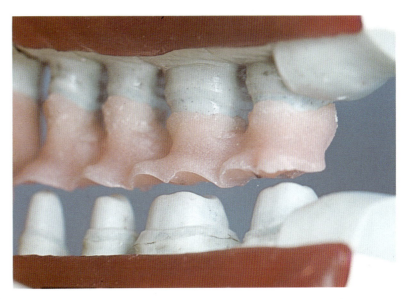

A lingual view of the right functonal guide.

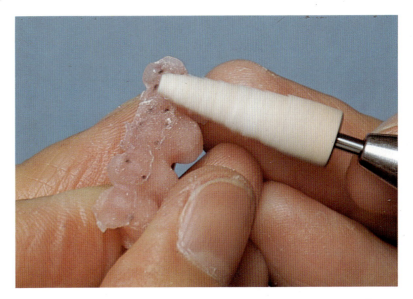

The margins of the functonal guides are finished with some extra fine sandpaper.

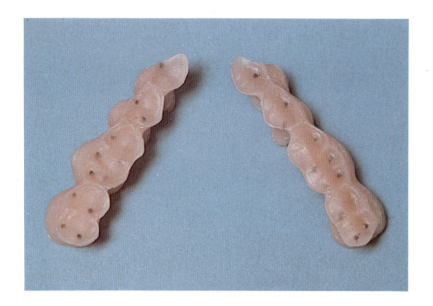

The finished right and left functional guides.

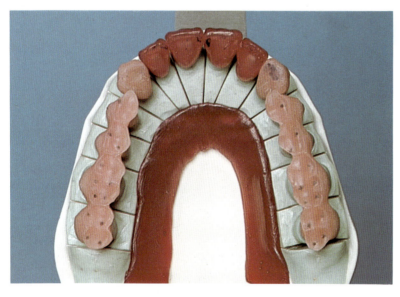

Occlusal view of the completed functional guides. The wax rod positions and other pertinent information are readily available.

Brief Summary: The present chapter presents the prerequisites for preparation of the occlusal surfaces for ceramometal restorations. The discussion covers the following:

1. The fabrication of planning wax crowns for the maxillary and mandibular anterior teeth.
2. The fabrication of silicone cores for the maxillary and mandibular anterior teeth.
3. The fabrication of maxillary and mandibular resin canines.
4. The fabrication of wax patterns of the mandibular anterior teeth.
5. The fabrication of functional guides.

In addition, reference is made to the construction of wax patterns for complete cast crowns for molars.

The author believes that the proper application of the skeletal technique enables a dental technician to construct a proper crown contour. The positioning of the cusps and the central fossae, using wax rods, has been illustrated as a technique useful in subsequent wax-ups. The significance of the resin canines is to ensure the correct vertical dimension between the dental arches. This method guarantees the strength of the anterior guidances during the entire wax-up. Silicone cores not only facilitate the fabrication of the resin canines, but also serve as reliable guides for subsequent procedures involving the addition of porcelain. The silicone cores also find application during the construction of the temporary crowns.

The functional guide proves to be valuable when the occlusal surfaces of the opposing tooth (teeth) are either defective or completely missing. When planning a porcelain restoration of any mandibular occlusal surface, the functional guide registers pertinent occlusal information. The proper utilization of the functional guide is indeed the key to the success of large scale restorations, including full mouth rehabilitation. In full mouth rehabilitation, where ceramometal restorations are utilized, it is imperative to observe all of the preliminary procedures discussed in this chapter. At first glance, these preliminary arrangements may seem inordinately complex, but they are absolutely necessary for the completion of high quality porcelain restorations.

The author wishes to emphasize that, instead of wasting time in a trial and error method, it is wiser to accept the methods discussed here, since they guarantee successful restorations through a series of sound and standardized step-by-step procedures.

4

FABRICATION OF THE PORCELAIN SUPPORTING METAL SUBSTRUCTURE

One of the main requirements for ceramometal restorations is strength. (The strength of both the metal alloy and porcelain, respectively, in addition to their combined strength.) In order to guarantee those properties, several conditions must be met.

The contour of the porcelain-supporting metal substructure is of prime concern, so the steps involved in the transition phase play a decisive role. Prevention of opaque exposure, adequate coloration, and functional crown contour are also greatly influenced by the transition phase. For the above reasons, the design of the wax coping and the adjustment of the ceramometal structure make the difference between success and failure of the final product. This chapter will discuss the step-by-step procedure for the ceramometal restoration.

4.1 THE CONCEPT OF TRIANGULAR STRUCTURE:

The retainer contour for a crown and bridge restoration is determined by its intended use and by the material used. In this section, the structural limitations of various materials are discussed. Special consideration is given to the marginal area of the abutment.

4.1.1. FOUR MAJOR REQUIREMENTS FOR THE CERAMOMETAL RESTORATION

The four major requirements for a successful ceramometal restoration are:
1. Proper condensation for maximum density.
2. Self-glazing rather than superficial glazing.
3. Incorporation of the porcelain coloration into the material, using the anatomical shading technique. The use of any kind of staining agent must be avoided in the cervical, proximal, papillary, and occlusal areas.
4. The opaque material must be concealed in order not to be exposed in the transition portion between the porcelain and the metal.

The composite of the constituent materials of the ceramometal crown: metal, porcelain, and opaque can be viewed as a triangle. Using this concept of triangular structure, the following is guaranteed:

A. The strength of the restoration

During the cementation of a ceramometal restoration, pressure is directed toward the restoration as indicated by the arrows (Fig. 4-1). In some cases, the metal becomes distorted and the porcelain cracks or exfoliates. In order to prevent this phenomenon, the ceramometal restoration must have sufficient strength. The creation of steps in the marginal region decreases the effect of pressure, thereby increasing the pressure-resistance of the material. At the same time, the combined strength of the metal and porcelain is enhanced.

B. The prevention of opaque exposure

Exposure of opaque material has been discussed in Chapter II, 1. Using the proper angle in the margin areas prevents this type of exposure (Fig. 4-4).

C. Proper porcelain coloration

The design of an adequate angle for the apex of the triangle structure guarantees sufficient thickness of the opaque, preventing the metallic color from showing through the porcelain material. This also provides the crown with the desired coloration, one closest to the natural color of the tooth. This is closely related to the problem of angulation of the abutment preparation, which will be discussed later.

D. The functional crown contour

The limitations of the constituent materials (metal, porcelain and opaque) must be understood in order to prevent overcontouring of the cervical region, and to guarantee a smooth transition to the root surface.

Fig. 4-1

The triangular structure of metal, opaque, and porcelain in the marginal portion of a chamfer type preparation.

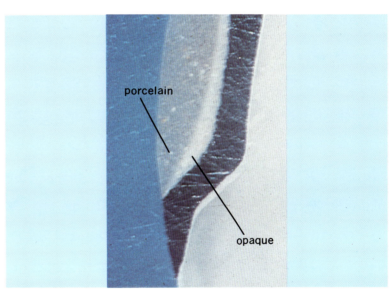

Direction of brush

Thickness of porcelain

metal (330μm)

opaque

Thickness of opaque

Opaque covered completely

Adequate strength will guarantee resistance to pressure

Sharp finish line

46μm

20μm

Fig. 4-2

The triangular concept in a bevel type preparation of the substructure (opaque and porcelain).

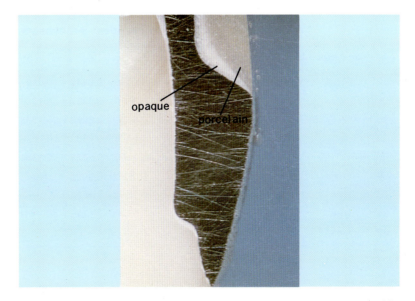

porcelain

opaque

Fig. 4-3

Triangular design of the supporting area (opaque and porcelain) — lingual view.

opaque   porcelain

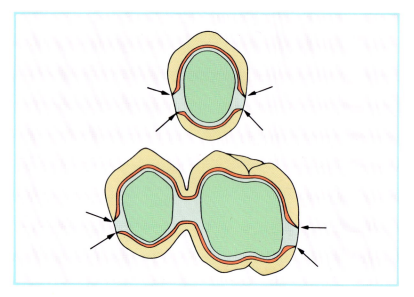

Fig. 4-4

The relationship of the three constituent materials in their mesial and distal aspects, viewed from the occlusal surface.

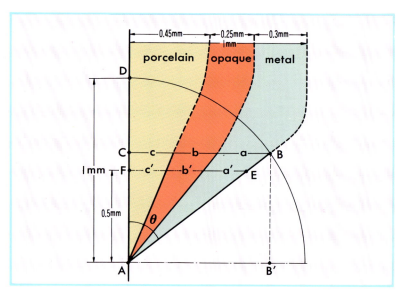

Fig. 4-5

A numerical scheme for the triangular structure.

Numerical values are dependent on changes in the angles in Fig. 4-5.

θ	a : metal	b : opaque	c : porcelain	a+b+c	AC	a′ : metal	b′ : opaque	c′ : porcelain	a′+b′+c′
10°	0.1736	0.	0	0.1736	0.9848	0.0881	0.	0	0.0881
20°	0.3	0.0420	0	0.3420	0.9397	0.1596	0.0223	0	0.1820
30°	0.3	0.2000	0	0.5000	0.8660	0.1732	0.1155	0	0.2887
40°	0.3	0.25	0.0928	0.6428	0.7660	0.1958	0.1632	0.0606	0.4196
50°	0.3	0.25	0.2160	0.7660	0.6428	0.2334	0.1945	0.1680	0.5958
60°	free	free	free	0.8660	0.5000	free	free	free	0.8660
70°	free	free	free	0.9397	0.3420	—	—	—	—
80°	free	free	free	0.9848	0.1736	—	—	—	—
90°	free	free	free	1.0000	0	—	—	—	—

(a+b+c=BC)　　　　　　　　　　　　　　　　(a′+b′+c′=EF)

4.1.2. THE NUMERICAL ANALYSIS OF THE TRIANGULAR STRUCTURE

The proper triangular structure — consisting of metal, opaque, and porcelain — determines how these metals are proportionately distributed. This determination is largely influenced by the angles and the width of the shoulder in the marginal region. Many factors play a role here, but they depend on the inherent limitations of the constituent materials. The formation of the apex of the triangle structure, covered by porcelain, must be based on a set of numerical calculations. The numerical values for the sides B and C of the upright triangle represent the respective thicknesses of the materials (Fig. 4-5).

a : A, metal thickness, 0.3 mm.
b : A, opaque thickness material, maximally 0.25 mm.
c : A, porcelain thickness over 0.2mm.

Point B, corresponding to the marginal angle B, is placed on the circumference of a circle with the radius AD. Thus we obtain the desired thickness from point A once the margin angle B is known. As a clinical guide, A is placed at 1mm beneath the gingival margin, which is difficult to manipulate in the dental laboratory. If it is possible to reproduce the position of A, the remaining tasks can be easily completed. Therefore, the segment BC indicates the necessary width which must be cut to form the triangle ABC. The segment AC refers to the height from the marginal apex. In this illustration, the average of the sum of the combined thicknesses of metal, opaque, and porcelain totals 1mm.

The reasons for assigning 0.3mm, 0.25mm, and 0.2mm to the respective constituent materials are listed below:

1. Metal thickness

Metal thickness varies according to the type of alloys used and the purpose of the prosthetic restoration. For instance, a complete crown requires a different metal thickness than a fixed partial denture. The margin of a metal restoration with a minimum thickness of 0.3mm has sufficient strength to withstand ordinary loading and is also strong enough to resist most forces encountered in dental laboratory procedures. When the gingival bevel happens to be shallow, we tend to render the metal thinner, possibly from 0.25mm down to 0.2mm, thoroughly reducing the strength of the restoration.

2. Opaque thickness

Opaque thickness has to be adjusted in each case, since the degree of its transparency depends on the composition of its ingredients. As a general consideration, it is desirable that its thickness be within a range of 0.1mm to 0.25mm. In some cases, a thickness of 0.18mm is sufficient to prevent the metal color from shining through the porcelain material.

3. Porcelain thickness

The minimum porcelain thickness is determined as 0.2mm. With porcelain thinner than 0.2mm, it is extremely difficult to cover marginal areas with porcelain.

The detemination of the correct thickness of opaque is dependent on the space provided for the porcelain in the marginal area. At present, margins are described variously as chamfers, shoulders, or bevels, but these terms usually do not indicate an angle. For this reason, the author divides the marginal angle into 90° in units of 10°, and employs the angle to determine the combination of constituent materials needed to then determine the necessary width of the bevel at a given angle.

1) The marginal angle is 10° (Fig. 4-6).

Only 0.1736mm are available for BC; the apex of the bevel will remain uncovered.

2) The marginal angle is 20° (Fig. 4-7).

0.3420mm is available, but when the thickness of the metal is subtracted from this value, the remaining width may be as little as 0.0420mm. This thickness is insufficient for proper porcelain coverage.

3) The marginal angle is 30° (Fig. 4-8).

Although 0.5mm is available on BC, after the subtraction of the metal thickness, the thickness for the opaque is insufficient.

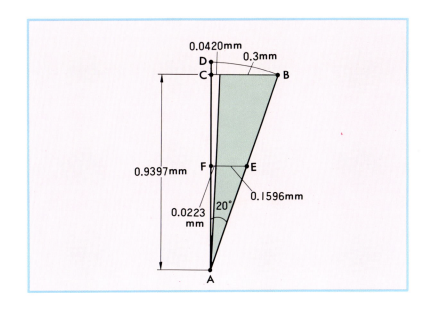

Fig. 4-6

Marginal angle of 10°

Fig. 4-7

Marginal angle of 20°

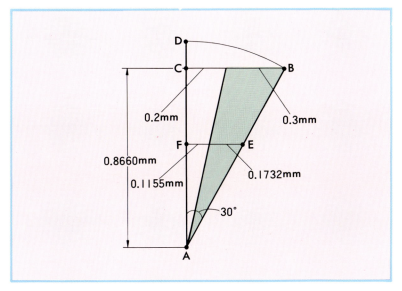

Fig. 4-8

Marginal angle of 30°

4) The marginal angle is 40° (Fig. 4-9).

Here again, the necessary porcelain thickness will be 0.0928mm. After both the metal and opaque thickness are subtracted, the marginal portion has to be finished with metal.

5) The marginal angle is 50° (Fig. 4-10).

When the apex of the margin A is placed 1mm beneath the gingiva, there will be 0.3572mm available, which roughly corresponds to a combined thickness of 0.75mm. Therefore, 0.2160mm of porcelain can cover the 0.3mm thick metal and the 0.25mm thick opaque. From these comparisons, we understand that 50° is the angle for the marginal portion. This is called the **critical angle.** The critical angle for the porcelain and opaque is about 35°.

6) The marginal angle is 60° (Fig. 4-11, 4-12).

The thickest possible metal portion is the triangle ZAX, and since Z can be changed, we are given more latitude for adjustments than with an angle of 50°.

7) The marginal angles are 70°, 80°, and 90° (Fig. 4-13 to 4-18).

As the angles of the marginal areas increase, the area within the triangle increases, along with the space available for adjustments. This facilitates the laboratory procedures. Thus we are able to guarantee a suitable width for the metal, porcelain, and opaque at the apex.

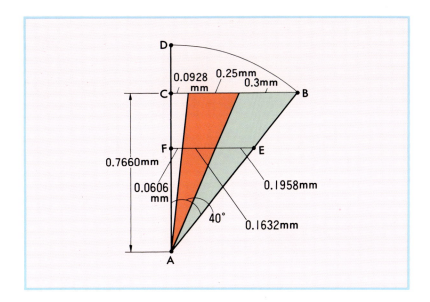

Fig. 4-9

Marginal angle of 40°.

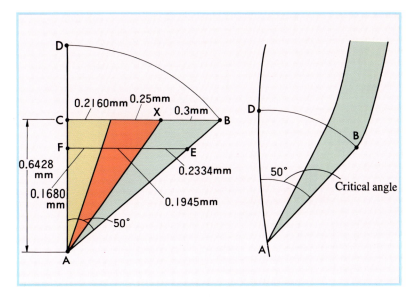

Fig. 4-10

The triangular structure at the 50° marginal angle, called the critical angle.

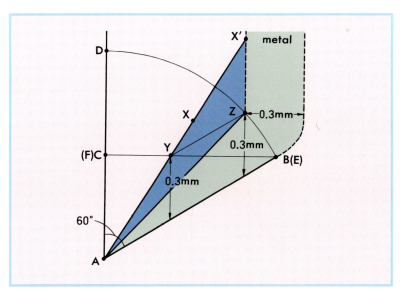

Fig. 4-11

A 60° marginal angle (the range of adjustment △AZX').

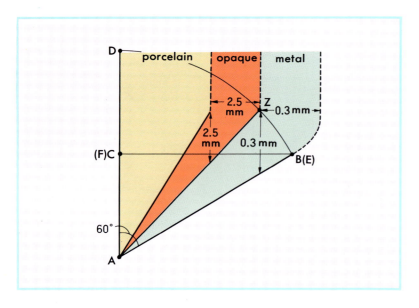

Fig. 4-12

The triangular structure at the 60° marginal angle (the range of adjustment △AZX').

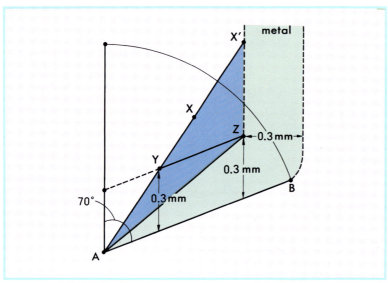

Fig. 4-13

A 70° marginal angle (the range of adjustment △AZX').

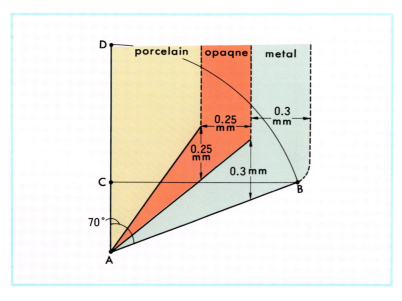

Fig. 4-14

A 70° marginal angle. The triangular structure at the 70° angle.

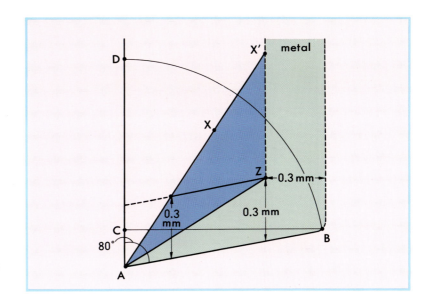

Fig. 4-15

The metal adjustment range at the 80° marginal angle (△AZX').

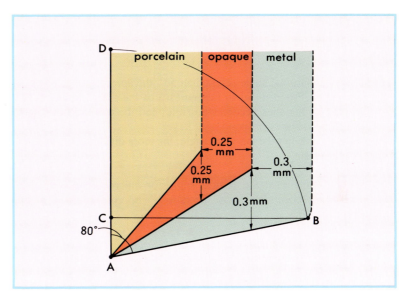

Fig. 4-16

The triangular structure at the 80° marginal angle, with the smallest possible angle for the metal portion.

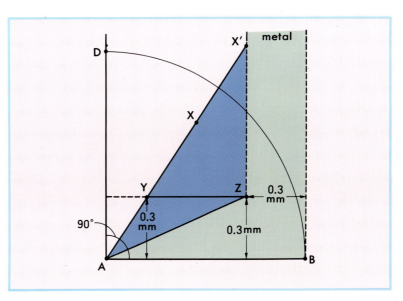

Fig. 4-17

The range adjustment at 90° (△AZX').

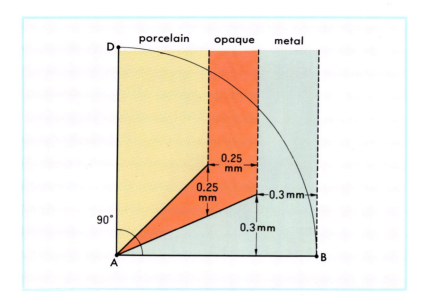

Fig. 4-18

The triangular structure at the marginal angle of 90°.

Summary:

1. When the marginal angle is less than 50°, the apex has to be finished with metal. Proportional to the increase of the marginal angle, the coverage of the apex becomes possible, and the room for the metal portion becomes correspondingly larger.

Inversely, the smaller the marginal angle, the more difficult the finishing of the metal portion.

2. In our calculations, the critical angle for the metal, opaque, and porcelain is postulated at 50° because of the convex shape of the clinical crown.

3. When the marginal angle is increased beyond 50°, the technician is given more leeway in his work and can select the appropriate width for each material.

4.1.3. THE TRIANGULAR STRUCTURE AND ITS SUPPORT AREA

The support area provides the transition area from the porcelain to the metal structure. It is necessary to guarantee a uniform layer of porcelain, so that the pressure exerted on the porcelain will be absorbed. This also serves to reinforce the porcelain, i.e. the support area corresponds to the metal structure, and the opaque and porcelain forms the angle of the support area. Proper establishment of this angle is important in order to provide the desired structure for the ceramometal restoration.

1. The support area is defined as the space where the porcelain covers the marginal apex.

In a proper restoration, the porcelain covers the margin without exposing any opaque, and the marginal angle has to be between 50° to 90°. If the marginal angle were prepared at 70°, the largest possible area would be $\triangle$ABX' and the smallest possible area would be $\triangle$ABZ with a metal thickness of 0.3mm (Fig. 4-19). As illustrated on the following pages, the area occupied by metal ranges from the minimum $\triangle$ABZ to the maximum AZX' and therefore, we may regard AZX' as "the range of possible adjustment."

When the metal portion is enlarged, we obtain a corresponding increase in strength. In practice, we use the minimum $\triangle$ABZ in which sufficient strength of the metal can be guaranteed. The adjustment of the supporting areas per se, including the selection of proper stones and burs, and the modification of their contour will be discussed later in this text.

2. The marginal support area with exposed metal.

When the marginal angle of the abutment is less than 50°, it is difficult to cover the tip of the margin with porcelain without exposing the opaque at the metal and containing an overcontour.

For this reason, metal will have to be exposed at an angle of less than 50°. In this situation, the angle of the support area, which contains the opaque and the porcelain, will have a critical angle of 35°. It is possible to reduce the amount of exposed metal at the margin, but this causes the angle of the support area to become too acute. The compressive occlusal load will thus be exerted on the porcelain. However with an obtuse angle, the great advantage is the combination of opaque material and porcelain (Fig. 4-22).

The supporting area of a metal restoration is within the range of the minimum $\triangle ABZ$ and the maximum $\triangle ABX'$. For this reason, $\triangle AZX'$ serves as a limitation for the adjustment (Fig. 4-23). When the metal area is enlarged, the metal strength can be increased correspondingly. Inversely, when the area is small, strength is gained in the supporting area.

During the preparation of an abutment tooth with an angle less than 50°, it is difficult to cover the marginal tip with porcelain without exposing the opaque or overcontouring the restoration. Therefore, when the marginal angle is less than 50°, the metal will have to be exposed. When the critical angle is set at 35°, the exposed portion of the metal is reduced at the margin, but its resistance against outside pressure is correspondingly weaker, because the angle of the supporting area is too abrupt. This influences the esthetic appearance of the anterior teeth. In practice, the metal coping is contoured to incorporate **a** and is covered with the opaque so that the periphery (**A**) can be covered with porcelain (Fig. 4-24).

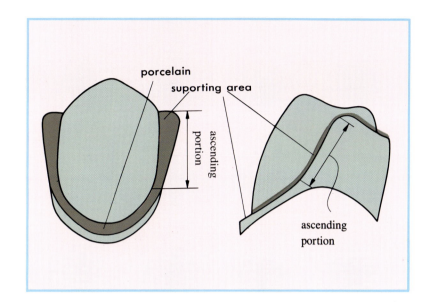

Fig. 4-19

This view shows the supporting area of the substructure.

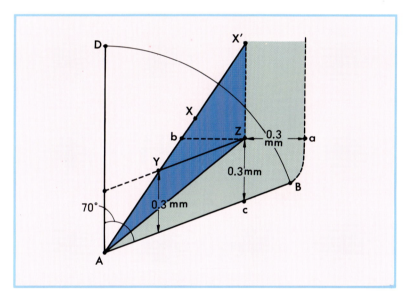

Fig. 4-20

The marginal angle is 70° (△AZX′).

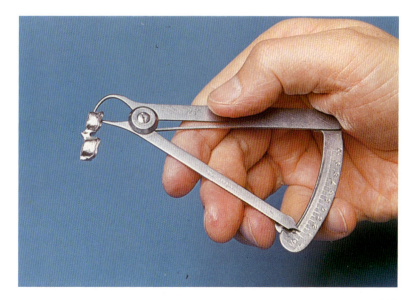

Fig. 4-21

A measurement of the porcelain thickness is made for the adjustment range of the support area.

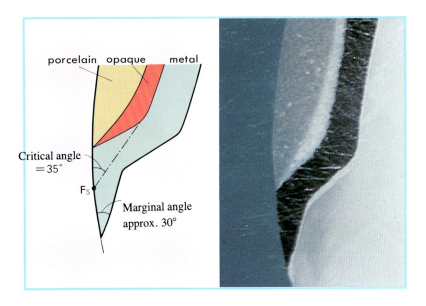

Fig. 4-22

The combination of opaque material and porcelain has a maximum angle of about 35°.

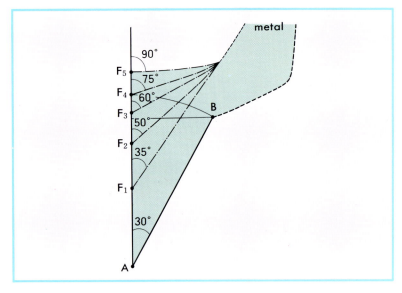

Fig. 4-23

A range of critical angles from 35° (F₁) to 90° (F₅). The amount of exposed metal is correlated with these angles. At F₁ the amount of exposed metal is minimal, increasing as we go up the scale, as illustrated.

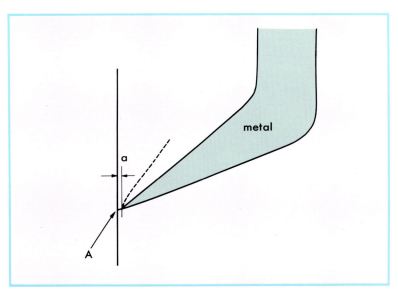

Fig. 4-24

For clinical purposes, the tip is covered with porcelain to the thickness of the penciled line.

4.2 MORPHOLOGICAL REQUIREMENTS FOR THE METAL SUBSTRUCTURE

One of the essential requirements for ceramometal restorations, the supporting structures provide a foundation for the contour, strength, and surface finish of the porcelain crown.

We must have a clear understanding of the requirements discussed in Chapter II in order to arrive at a physiological and esthetically satisfactory restoration. In the following text, we will discuss some of the basic principles governing these complex techniques.

4.2.1 BASIC REQUIREMENTS

The major requirement for the successful ceramic restoration is a uniform thickness of the porcelain in connection with the underlying metal structure. Attention must be directed to that fact, because porcelain has low tensile strength and elasticity. Unless it is properly supported, it wll not withstand masticatory forces. Fig. 4-25 illustrates this quite well: a uniform layer of porcelain is fired onto a metal ball and thus supported, so sufficient strength of the porcelain and compressive bonding is obtained. When restoring a crown with a ceramometal casting, the porcelain is built up heavily on the cusp tips, but is thin in the marginal areas. Therefore, it is difficult to obtain uniform porcelain thickness. When the disparity in porcelain thickness exceeds a certain limit, exfoliation is likely to occur from occlusal loading. The fracture of the porcelain is most frequently encountered in the cervical region, cusp tip areas, and other weak portions of the restoration. The restoration must have a certain minimum porcelain thickness in all areas in order to withstand occlusal forces.

1) The proper contour to guarantee structural compressive bonding.

Structural compressive bonding entails the metal support of the porcelain. This is illustrated in Figs. 4-26 and 4-27. A metal structure covered completely with porcelain increases its structural compressive bonding and, through the increased surface area, both chemical and mechanical bonding are also improved. Ideally, this type of structure should have a rounded shape and the incline on the lingual surface must be contoured carefully. If the metal structure is contoured like Fig. 4-28 or Fig. 4-29, satisfactory bonding cannot be guaranteed, since the restoration will be exposed to detrimental stresses. The porcelain may then fracture, being unable to withstand lateral forces.

2) The ideal resistance form to withstand occlusal forces.

The concept of resistance form derives from the fact that a broad curve allows the construction of an even surface (Fig. 4-30). It is apparent that a metal structure with a wide surface can easily withstand occlusal stresses and other forces exerted on it from different angles (Fig. 4-31). The concept of reinforcing the bases of the incisal and cuspal areas with metal is also important when we are dealing with vertical occlusal forces representing compressive loading (Fig. 4-32). The support area of the metal substructure has the purpose of converting the occlusal forces exerted on the porcelain into a compressive force (Fig. 4-33).

3) The ideal contour to withstand distortional forces directed onto the porcelain.

We recall that the larger the base of the triangle, the more effectively it can deal with any force exerted on its sides. When we compare the incisal or cuspal area with a triangle, we can easily understand that, if this area has a wide enough base, it can better counteract any lateral force.

As illustrated in Fig. 4-34, the proper angle of the supporting area has the same basis in the theory of triangle structure (Fig. 4-35).

4) Ideal contour without partial concentration of occlusal forces.

If a pronounced convex area is created on any portion of the fired porcelain surface, occlusal forces are partially concentrated on the convex area (Fig. 4-36). This may lead to porcelain fracture. A piece of glass can be more easily cut into sections when it is given sharp notches rather than obtuse ones.

5) Porcelain contour with localized shrinkage.

When a convex spot is on the surface of a porcelain object, there is a disparity in thickness which leads to uneven firing. As illustrated in Fig. 4-36, shrinkage tends to take place in the direction of the arrow and is one of the causes of porosities and cracks between the junction of the porcelain and the metal alloy.

6) The ideal contour to guarantee a smooth finish of contacts and occlusal surfaces.

During the preparation of teeth for any ceramometal restoration, we apply a basic principle: a junction between the porcelain and metal must be avoided in areas where the restoration contacts opposing and/or adjacent teeth. The heterogenous materials metal, opaque, and porcelain used here constitute a multiphased restoration compared with a single phased restoration. Using either metal alloy or porcelain, the same degree of surface finish is more difficult to achieve in a multiphasic restoration. This is also valid for any minute adjustments which may be required in the oral cavity. It is important that the angle of the supporting proximal area be large enough, with its rise positioned lingually, and that the contact areas be built up with a single phased material.

In some cases, it is necessary to establish a contact area between the opposing teeth in violation of the above principle. The angle of the supporting area and the combination of the opaque and porcelain must be given careful consideration (Fig. 4-37). In such a situation, the supporting area must be prepared at an obtuse angle and the use of opaque omitted. Thus, we avoid exposing the opaque material during occlusal adjustment. Because of the almost 180° degree angle of the supporting area, the metal color can be kept to a minimum.

7) The contour compensating for deficiencies in the preparation of the abutment tooth.

When the abutment is too short and there is not enough mesiodistal reduction, an uneven distribution of the porcelain can often be observed (Fig. 4-38). Porcelain is a very hard material, yet is easily subjected to fractures by impact or other forces when not properly supported. In the case of a very short abutment, elective endodontic treatment is carried out and a metal core can be used to compensate for that problem. The metal core must be contoured accordingly. When adequate retention and strength of the restorations remain questionable, even if several teeth are used as abutments, we can employ some other means to evenly distribute the occlusal forces.

One solution for the above problem would be to include several abutments in the fixed partial denture in order to reinforce the final restoration or, in some cases, to remove one or several abutment teeth from the group function design and reduce the cuspal inclination angle in order to relieve lateral pressure.

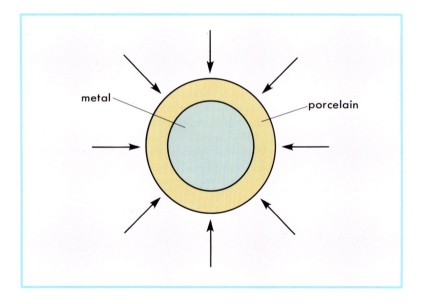

Fig. 4-25

When a metal ball is coated with an even thickness of porcelain, we can create adequate structural compressive bonding.

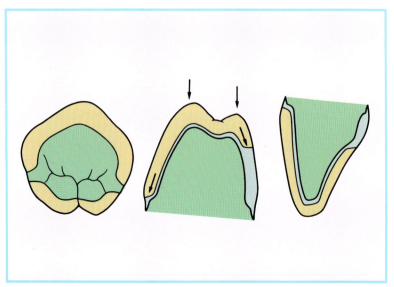

Fig. 4-26

In order to obtain adequate strength, it is necessary to coat the metal core with an even layer of porcelain.

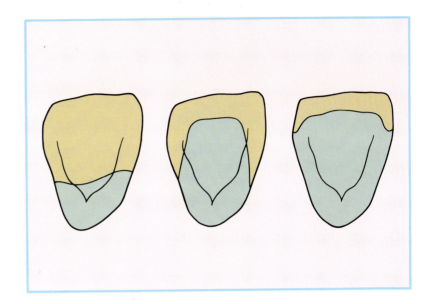

Fig. 4-27

The distribution of metal and porcelain in well designed anterior restorations.

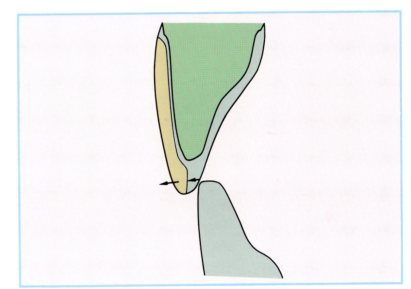

Fig. 4-28

This design of a metal core will fracture easily.

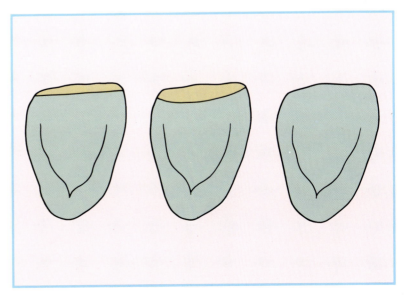

Fig 4-29

Another example of an inadequately designed metal core.

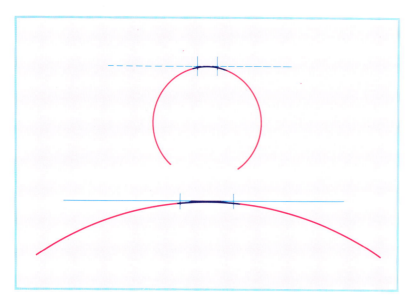

Fig 4-30

A wide curve guarantees an even and wide surface for our purposes.

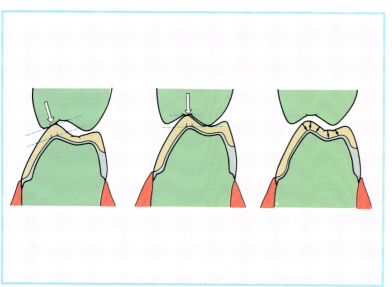

Fig. 4-31

This design can compensate for occlusal forces exerted from different angles.

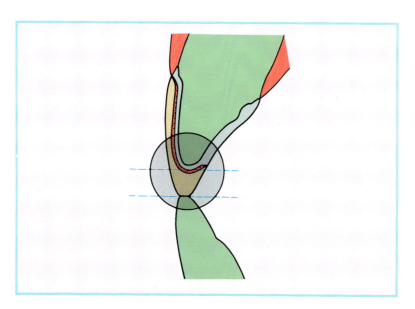

Fig. 4-32

This design of the metal core is rounded at the incisal region. During edge-to-edge contact, the incisal edges of the opposing teeth are brought parallel to each other as much as possible, so that the occlusal forces may be evenly distributed.

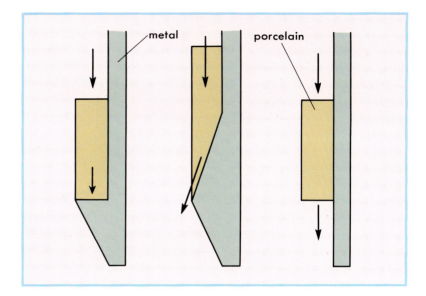

Fig. 4-33

Establishing a supporting area and providing an adequate angle for it are very important in compensating for occlusal loading.

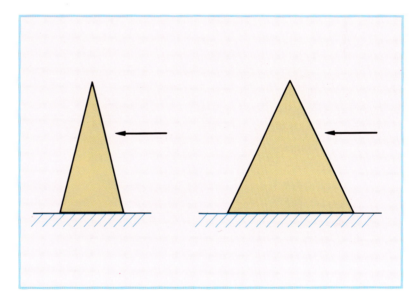

Fig. 4-34

A larger base can counteract lateral force more effectively.

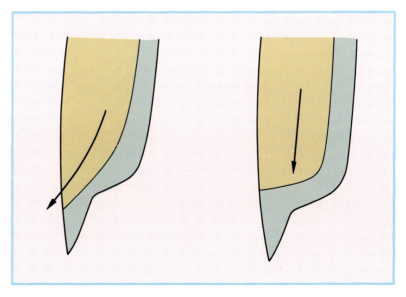

Fig. 4-35

The angles of the supporting area are important: they have to resist forces from various directions.

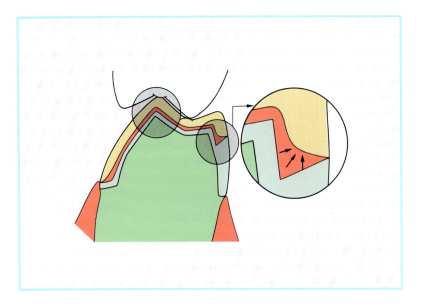

Fig. 4-36

If a convex area exists on the surface of the metal core, forces tend to partially concentrate on it. This may result in the fracture of the porcelain. Moreover, it may lead to the formation of porosities and cracks.

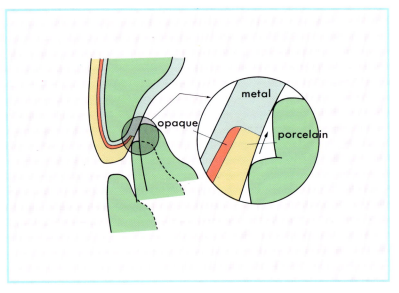

Fig. 4-37

When it is necessary to establish a supporting area in the protrusive path between the opposing teeth, it must be prepared at a very obtuse angle approximating 180°. The application of opaque is then omitted.

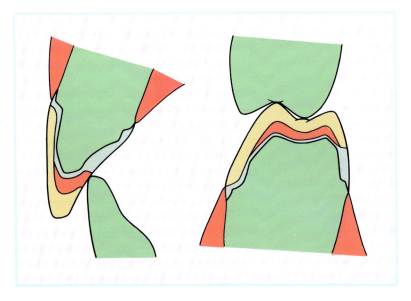

Fig. 4-38

The design of a metal core on an unsatisfactory (too short) abutment.

4.2.2 ESTABLISHING THE SUPPORT AREAS

The morphological requirements of the metal core have been discussed in paragraph 4.2. In addition to those requirements, another one is the provision of supporting areas in the inclines of the labial, buccal and lingual surfaces and in the proximal regions.

With the proper combination of the metal, opaque, and porcelain constituents and their application in thin layers, we try to accomplish the following objectives.

1. Sufficient strength
2. Smooth surface finish and prevention of opaque exposure
3. Proper coloration of the porcelain
4. Creation of functional contour

The angulation of the supporting area determines whether the crown margin is covered with crown porcelain or is largely exposed. The angle of 50° is generally considered necessary in order to cover the margin with crown porcelain. The supporting areas affects the following:

1. The strength of the metal alloy in the supporting area
2. The combination of opaque and porcelain in the supporting area
3. The translation of occlusal loading on the porcelain into compressive forces, in addition to the ability of the porcelain to withstand distortion

The inclines of the proximal supporting areas are also closely related to the labial (buccal) and lingual areas. The provision of a supporting area is a basic requirement for the planning and execution of the ceramometal restoration. Our understanding of the principles discussed above guarantees successful restoration.

4.2.3 THE CONTOUR OF THE SOLDER JOINT (RIGID CONNECTOR)

The maintenance of oral hygiene is important and largely depends on the positioning of the teeth and the positioning and size of their proximal contacts and embrasures. Oral hygiene is even harder to accomplish when prosthetic devices are to be cared for. When crowns or bridges are connected, we must be concerned about their conjoint strength and about the maintenance of the patient's oral health. In order to ensure the best oral hygiene, small connectors are more desirable than wide ones, if strength can be guaranteed simultaneously. The ideal contour of the solder joint must provide the following:

1. When viewed labially or lingually, the solder joint must be sufficiently strong while still providing for easy maintenance of oral hygiene (Fig. 4-39a, 39b).
2. From a mesial or distal view, the rigid connector angles should be obtuse, creating a junction in the form of an inverted triangle, which will guarantee the necessary strength. The overall rounded contour of the solder joint increases strength and improves oral hygiene (Fig. 4-39c).
3. When viewed from the alveolar ridge area, the angles must be obtuse, never acute. The base of the solder joint must be wide for both strength and maintenance of oral hygiene (Fig. 4-40).
4. The gingival contour of the solder joint:
    a. It shall not impinge on the interdental papillae and adjacent gingivae.
    b. Contact with the interdental papillae and gingivae is kept to a minimum and the embrasures are contoured in order to facilitate cleansing measures and to aid in selfcleansing.
5. The occlusal portion of the solder joint:
    a. The occlusal surfaces must be correctly contoured anatomically to guarantee proper function and esthetics.
    b. With sufficient crown length, the occlusal portion of the solder joint can be placed adjacent to the occlusal half of the prepared tooth.
    c. In the absence of sufficient crown length, the necessary strength can be obtained by placing the occlusal portion of the solder joint higher than the occlusal surface of the abutment (Fig. 4-42).

These theoretical considerations direct our decisions. Often we are confronted with more involved situations when opposing teeth and the functional guides are partially or completely missing.

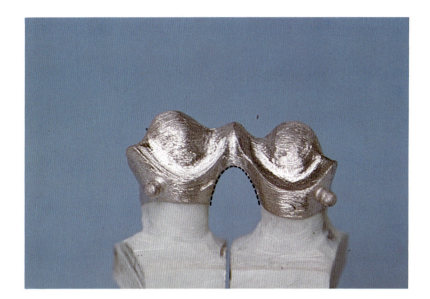

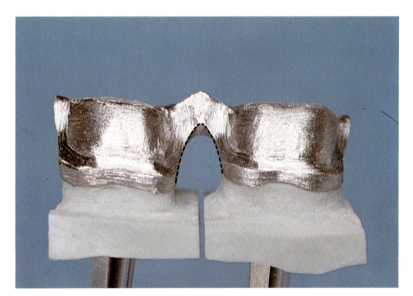

Fig. 4-39a, b

Using a trestle design in the solder joint, we can obtain greater strength and arrive at a satisfactory contour for the embrasures.

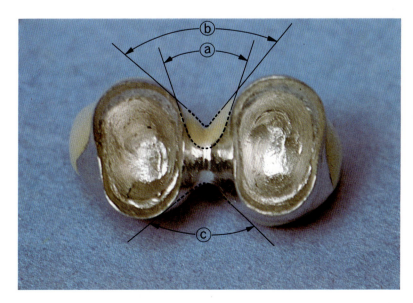

Fig. 4-39c

In the solder joint, sections ⓐ and ⓒ are given a globular appearance and angles ⓐ, ⓑ, and ⓒ are rendered as wide as possible for the purpose of both the guarantee of strength and maintenance of oral hygiene.

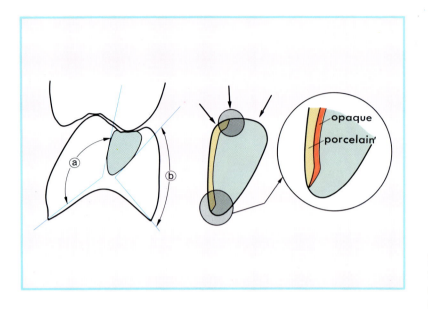

Fig. 4-40

In the mesio-distal section, the solder joint has the shape of an inverted triangle with rounded corners. The angles between **a** and **b** are rendered wide enough to guarantee strength and to facilitate proper oral hygiene.

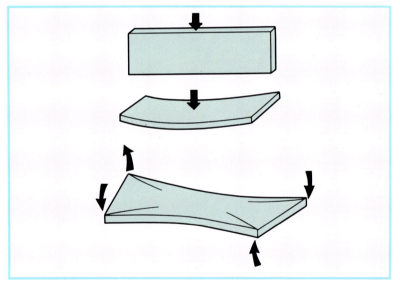

Fig. 4-41

When planning the contour of the rigid connector, any warping or distortion of the solder assembly must be prevented.

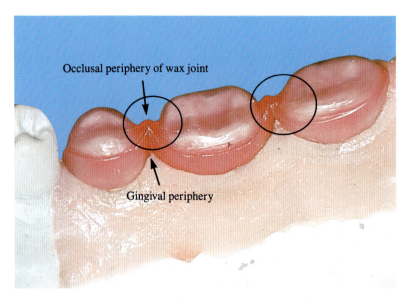

Fig. 4-42

Here the occlusal periphery of the wax joint is extended beyond the height of the abutment in order to guarantee sufficient strength.

4.2.4 PONTIC CONTOUR

The pontic contour must fulfill the requirements mentioned in the preceding text. In addition, the following must be observed:

1. The base portion in contact with the oral mucosa is prepared from either metal or porcelain, and the junction between the metal and porcelain is placed away from the underlying mucosa (Fig. 4-43, 4-44).
2. Any area which is in contact with the opposing teeth is covered with either porcelain over metal or metal alone (Fig. 4-43, 4-44).
3. The shape of the pontic must facilitate the maintenance of oral hygiene (Fig. 4-45, 46).
4. The contour of the solderjoint and the metal core must be planned carefully in order to increase strength. It is important to design them properly to resist the vertical direction of occlusal forces (Fig. 4-47).

Fig. 4-43

Improper design: the ceramometal junction is in contact with the oral mucosa.

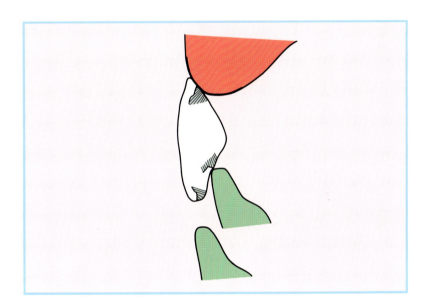

Fig. 4-44

Another improper design: the ceramometal junction is in contact with the oral mucosa and the occlusal surfaces of the opposing teeth.

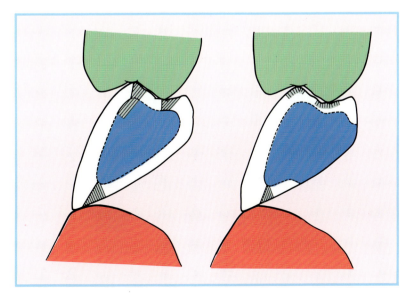

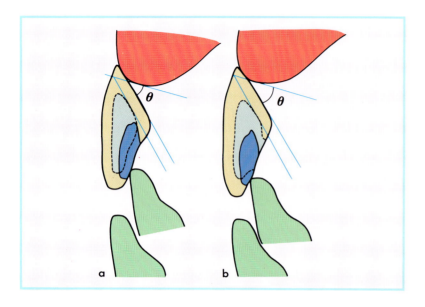

Fig. 4-45

Correct design for anterior pontics. The grey area indicates the metal coping; the blue outlines the solder joint.

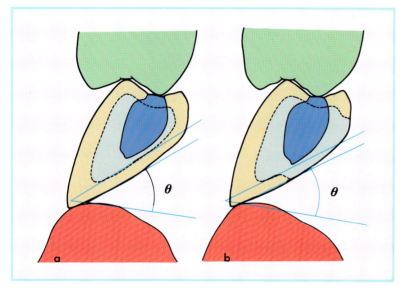

Fig. 4-46

Correct design for molar pontics. The grey color indicates the metal; the blue outlines the solder joint.

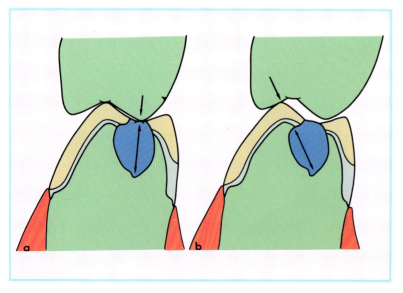

Fig. 4-47

The occlusal load is directed vertically as indicated by arrows (a). It is directed sideways during mastication and lateral excursions (b).

4.3 FABRICATION OF THE WAX PATTERN FOR THE SUBSTRUCTURE

When performing full mouth rehabilitation with ceramometal restorations, the following steps must be observed:

1. Diagnostic wax-ups of the maxillary and mandibular anterior teeth
2. Fabrication of silicone cores for the maxillary and mandibular anterior teeth
3. Fabrication of the maxillary and mandibular resin canines
4. Diagnostic wax-ups for the maxillary and mandibular molars
5. Fabrication of the functional guides

Only after completing these preliminary steps can wax-up of the metal coping begin.

Some of the preliminaries to the wax-up may appear to be a waste of time, but more accurate results are obtained by using sheet wax for the fabrication of the wax pattern. During routine tooth preparations for ceramometal restorations, the practitioner follows standardized procedures which provide for satisfactory reduction of tooth substance in order to guarantee proper thickness of the porcelain. To wax up the pattern for the coping, the practitioner must be familiar with the following:

1) Morphological requirements for the substructure
2) The theory of triangular structure
3) The three basic planes that constitute crown contour

In this connection, the soft gingiva model and the diagnostic wax-up provide the most important frames of reference.

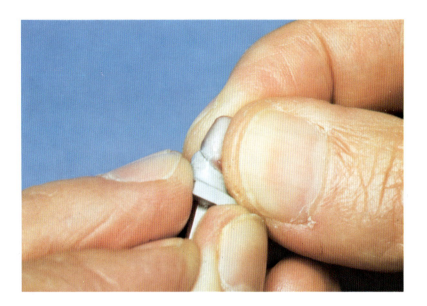

The first step of the crown wax-up consists of the adaptation of the sheet wax to the die. At the marginal area, the inlay wax is well adapted by using finger pressure. Since these copings will be cast in metal, their margins must be given particular attention. They should not be removed from the die until the practitioner is ready to invest the completed wax pattern.

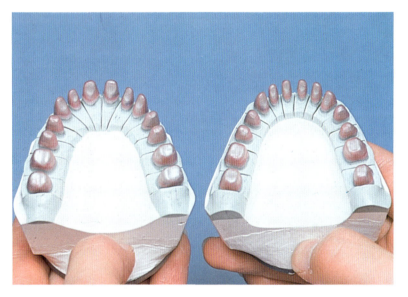

All maxillary and mandibular sub-structures completed.

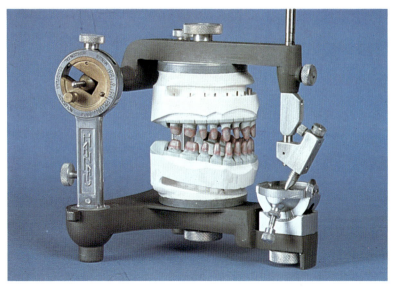

At this time, the maxillary and mandibular casts are mounted on the articulator.

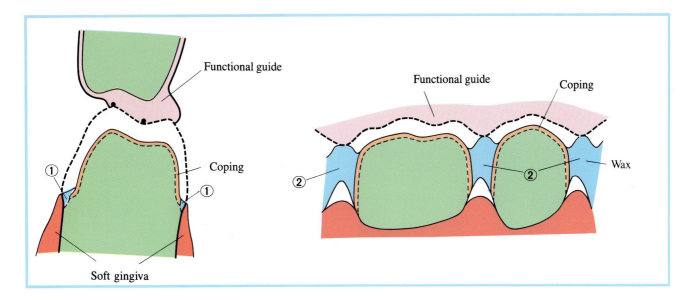

The thickness of the sheet wax is about 0.5mm. Now more wax is added on the coping to produce the final wax pattern. Frames of reference are added to the soft gingiva and planning crown, and functional guides are established for the mandibular molars. The margin is refined and the proximal portions of the copings are linked buccolingually in the center.

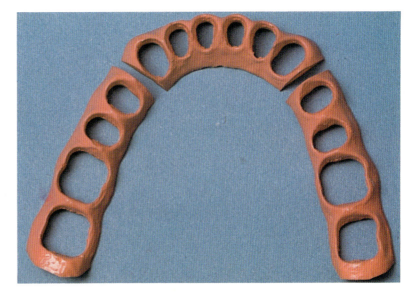

The soft gingiva is prepared and cut into three small sections. Here the cuts are placed between the canine and premolars, but they may also be placed at each papilla, if necessary.

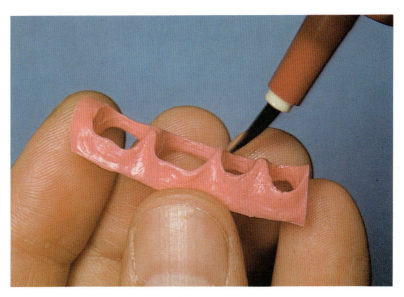

Prior to waxing up, a thin coat of a separator is applied to the inner surface of the three gingival parts of the soft gingiva.

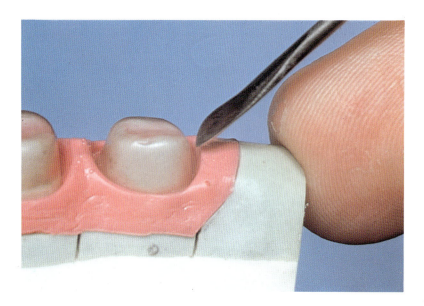

Wax is added in the space between the soft gingiva and the die margin to close it.

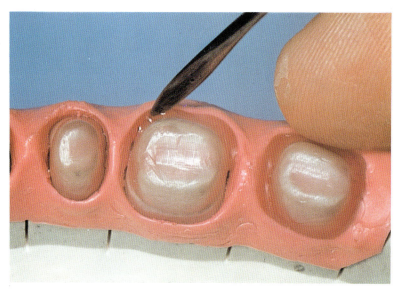

The wax needs to be properly melted in order to flow easily into minor crevices.

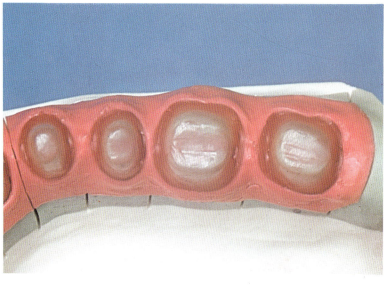

By closing this space, the proper marginal thickness and foundation for the later contour can both be obtained. Thus the guide for preparation of the wax pattern is also obtained.

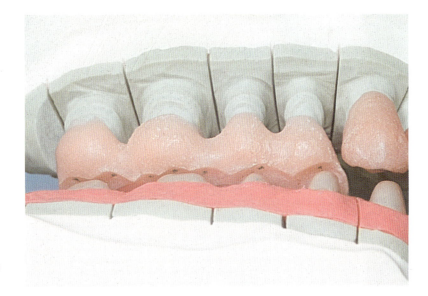

With reference to the soft gingiva, the interdental papillae are prepared.

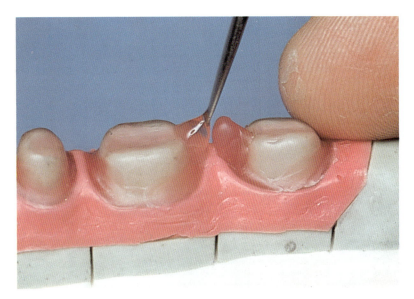

Contact areas and junctions of the proximal molar portions are waxed up next. To begin with, the proximal portions are prepared and the maxillary and mandibular limits are established in reference to the functional guide. The mesial side of one tooth and the distal side of the adjacent tooth are alternately waxed up, and the cusp ridges are joined.

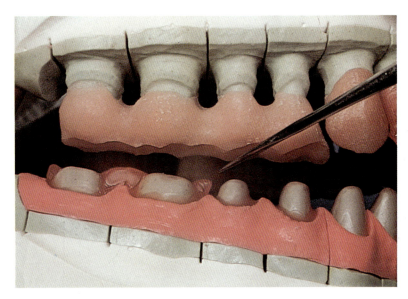

The preparation of the proximal contour is carried out on the articulator within the guidelines established. The functional guide is always uscd, the soft gingiva employed only when needed.

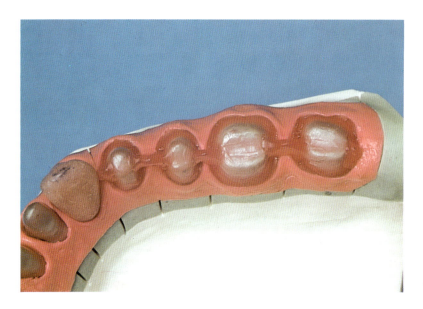

When preparing the proximal contour, the buccolingual center is used as a guideline.

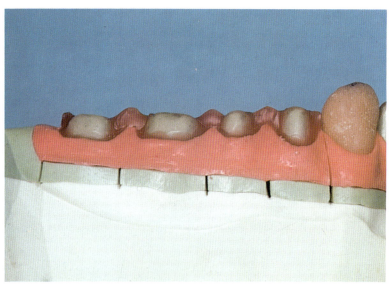

The buccal view of the mandibular right molars is used as a criterion for the preparation of the proximal contour.

The mandibular molars only are joined, the rest of the teeth remaining unconnected, but all the proximal spaces are filled in with wax so that this portion of the dental arch is treated as one entity. The proximal areas serve as necessary skeletons during subsequent procedures.

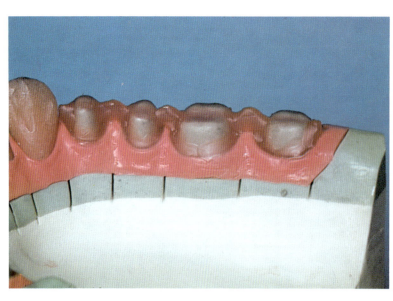

A lingual view. Vertical relations are established within the limits mentioned above.

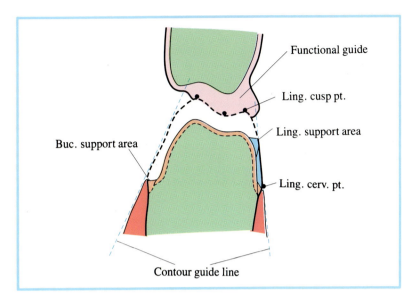

Because of the functional guide, the lingual cusp tips are already determined, giving a fairly good idea of the lingual cervical area. Thus, the surface contour of the mandibular molars can be anticipated. Furthermore, the thickness of the coping (0.5mm) enables the practitioner to decide where the supporting area must be placed with respect to the triangle structure (metal, opaque, and porcelain). When the vertical relationships of the supporting area are determined, the exposure area of the lingual metal is then finished and the buccal supporting area prepared.

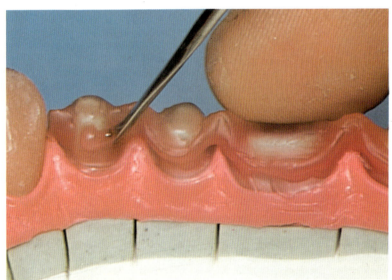

The area determining the vertical relations of the lingual supporting region is U-shaped. This U shape is the area where the metal portion has its maximum thickness. The diagnostic crown and the silicone core furnish useful information for this portion of the task.

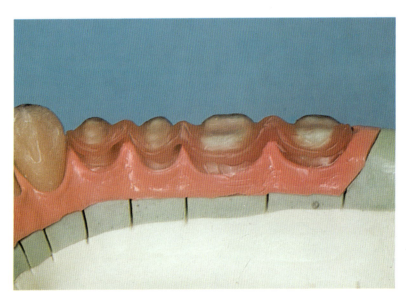

A view of the mandibular right molars in which the lingual supporting areas are completed. Notice the U-shaped skeletons.

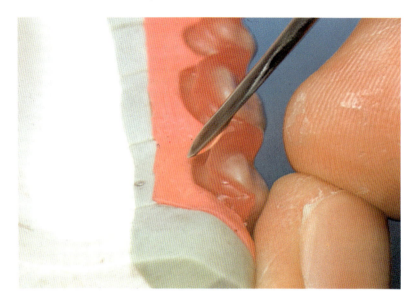

Next, the spaces between the lingual cervical portion and the supporting areas are filled in. As the wax sets in the spaces, the additional amount of wax necessary can be easily calculated.

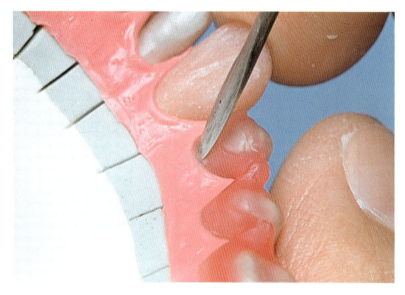

A carving instrument is placed along the lingual center from one tooth to the adjacent one to establish the proper arch contour in one step.

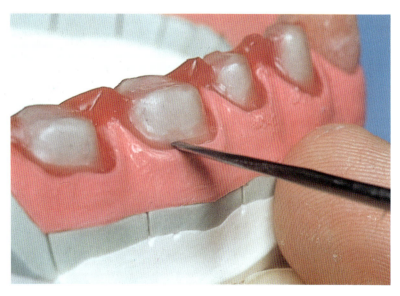

The supporting area is waxed up along the upper rim of the gingiva of the soft gingiva portion.

After completion of the wax-up, the proximal areas are cut into sections. Each tooth is removed from the model and minor modifications are made on the individual die.

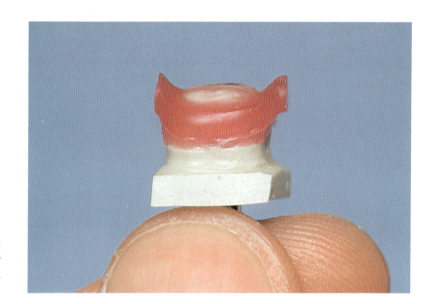

A mandibular first molar seen from the lingual side. The line on the upper rim of the gingival margin is clearly visible. An exposed lingual area is repaired. In this particular case, the margin is beneath the gingival rim and placed within the gingival sulcus.

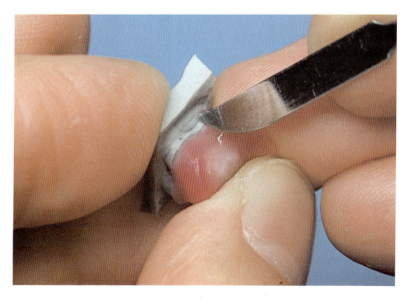

The result of an impression technique which exerts pressure on the gingiva.

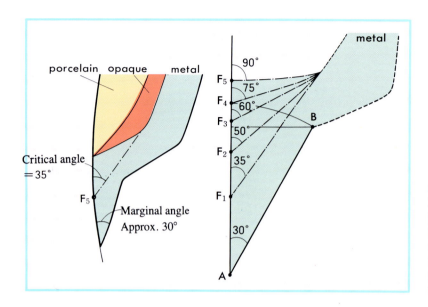

porcelain opaque metal

Critical angle
=35°

F₅

Marginal angle
Approx. 30°

90°

F₅ 75°
F₄ 60°
F₃
    50°
F₂ 35°

F₁

30°

A

B

metal

When the marginal angle is less than 50°, the final restoration will show exposed metal. In order to adhere to the triangular structure previously discussed, the critical angle is about 35°. In order to establish this structure, the angle of the supporting area ranges from 35° (F_1) to 90° (F_5), and the area of exposed metal increases as the angle increases from F_1 to F_5.

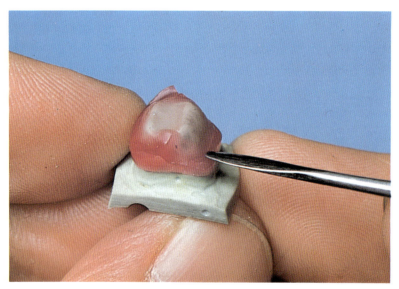

Here the buccal supporting area is adjusted in a continuous motion.

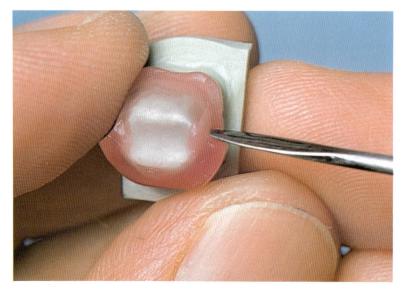

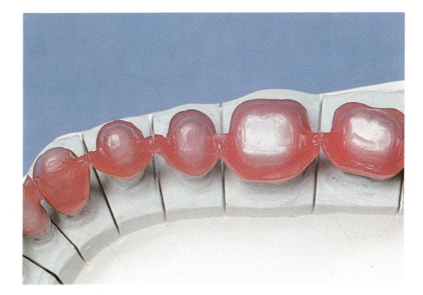

An occlusal view of the mandibular right molars. The positions of the buccolingual proximal supporting areas are now completed.

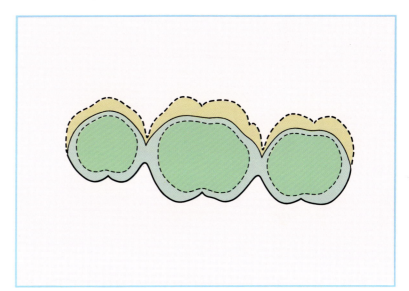

With this type of proximal contour, it is difficult to adequately cover the metal portion with uniformly thick porcelain. Therefore, this type of proximal contour must be avoided.

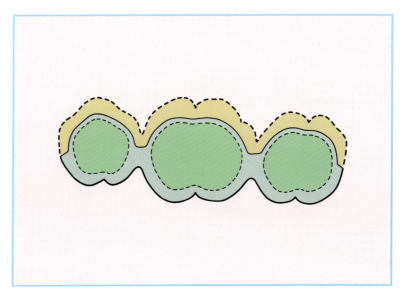

Here the ideal proximal contour is shown. The supporting area is positioned lingually on the mesial side of the second premolar. Contacts are established with the adjacent teeth.

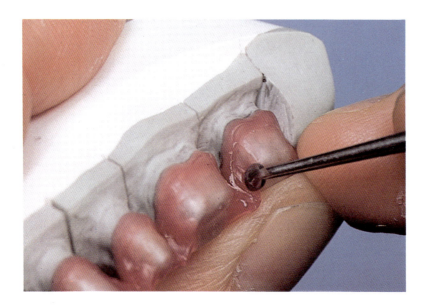

The proximal porcelain region must be as evenly contoured as possible. The supporting area is simultaneously established for the proximal region.

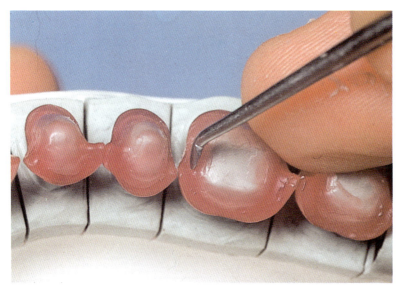

The distal surface of the second premolar and the mesial surface of the first molar are inclined somewhat lingually to facilitate joining them proximally with porcelain.

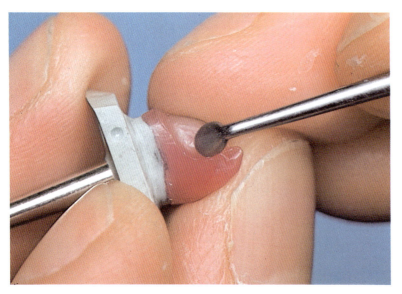

The wax crowns on the dies are removed from the model, and the buccal supporting areas are finished.

A heated Lekron instrument is recommended for this procedure, since it will not damage the surface of the copings. The same steps are repeated on the distal side.

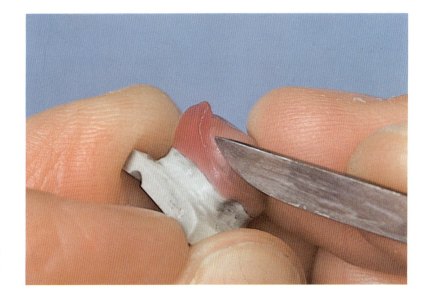

In the next step, the edge of a heated carving knife is used to adjust the transition from the supporting areas to the copings.

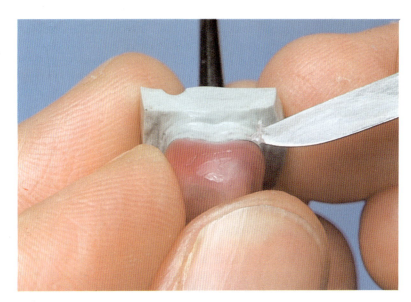

Thus, the molar wax pattern is almost completed.

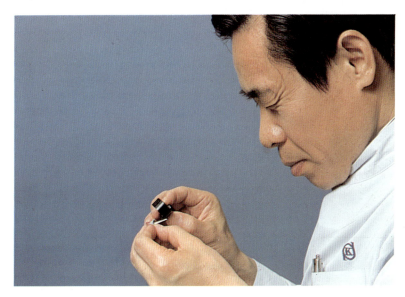

The marginal areas are carefully finished under magnification. (Either microscopic or stereo-telescopic magnification is recommended for this purpose.)

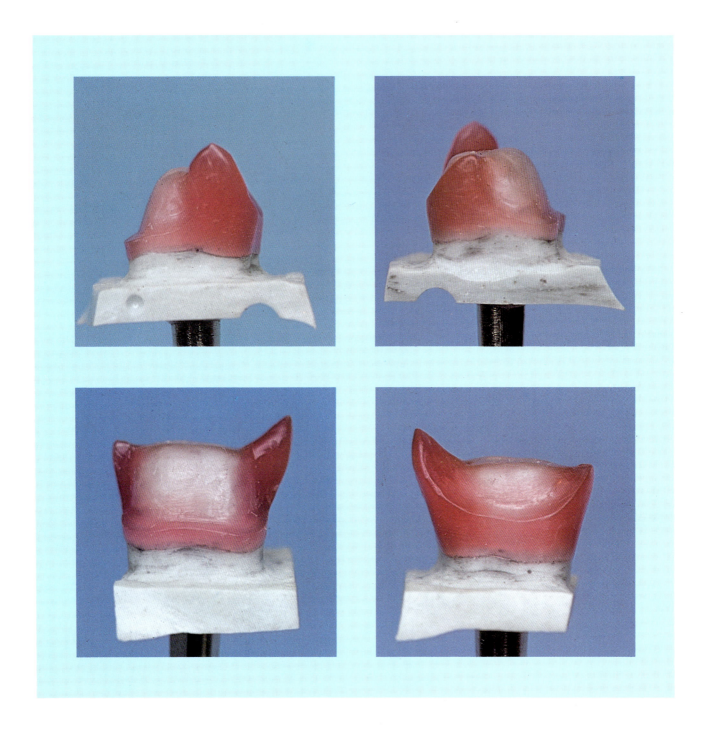

Left Above: A mesial view of the mandibular second molar wax
pattern.

Left Below: A buccal view of the same. The
mesial junctions show correct
vertical dimensions set up by
using the functional guides and
the soft gingiva.

Right Above: A distal view of the same.
Note the correct contour angulations of the supporting
areas.

Right Below: A lingual view of the same.
Note the wide supporting
area. This design will compensate for excessive occlusal
loading.

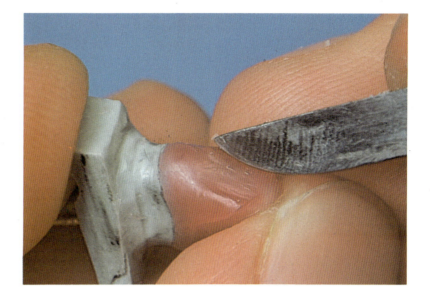

The wax patterns for the anterior teeth are constructed next. Basically, the technique is the same as shown on the molars. Here a heated carving knife is used to finish the lingual surface of a canine.

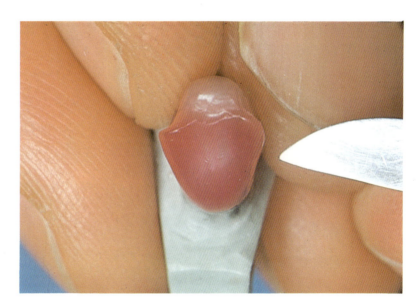

An incisal view of the canine wax pattern with an unfinished margin. By building up the porcelain in the supporting area as evenly as possible, no opaque is exposed. Moreover, when the canine cusp and incisal edges are contoured in a wide curvature, the porcelain can compensate effectively for vertical and/or lateral forces.

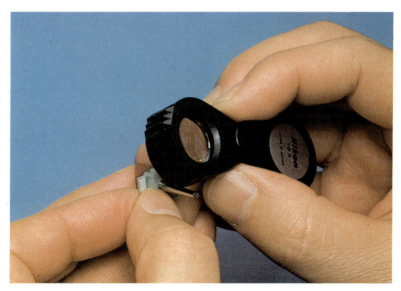

The wax pattern is examined under magnification.

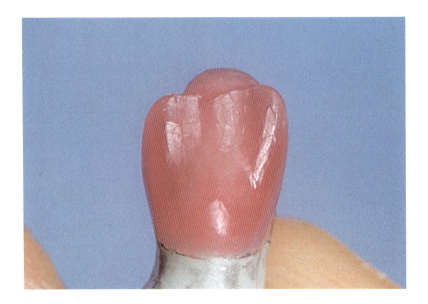

A lingual view of the maxillary canine wax pattern. The contour of the exposed metal is determined by the relationship between the surface, the tongue, and the flow of food particles.

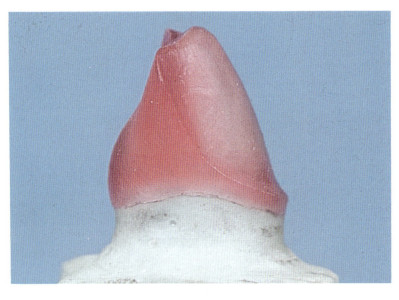

A distal view of the same.

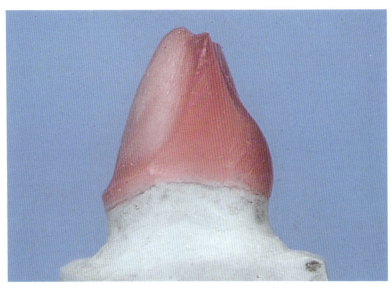

A mesial view of the same.

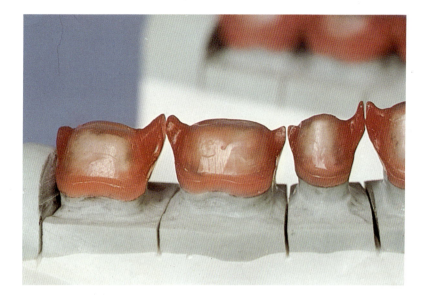

In this particular case, both the mandibular premolars and the molars are connected. This view of the mandibular molars shows the individual wax patterns.

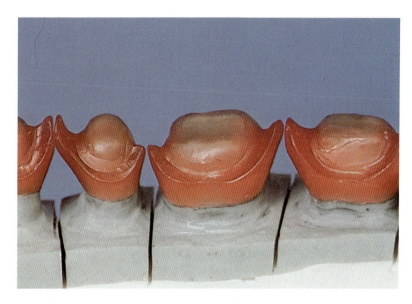

A lingual view of the same.

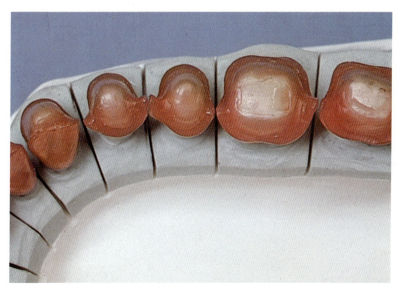

An occlusal view of the same; the junction is positioned buccolingually to the center.

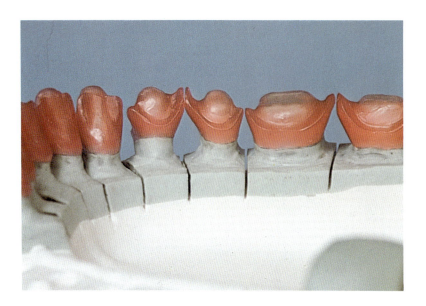

When connecting the wax patterns, it is extremely important to check that the dies and the plasterkey are correctly positioned.

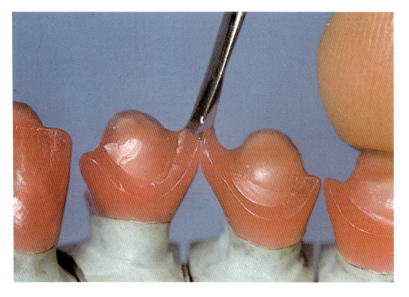

The first and second premolars are waxed together. The wax connector is constructed in archform and the gingival embrasures are contoured accordingly. This type of architectural bridge design guarantees strength sufficient to resist occlusal forces directed onto the teeth.

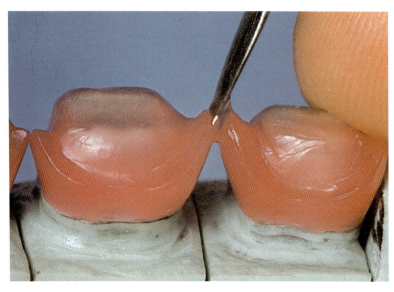

The first and second molars are joined in the same manner.

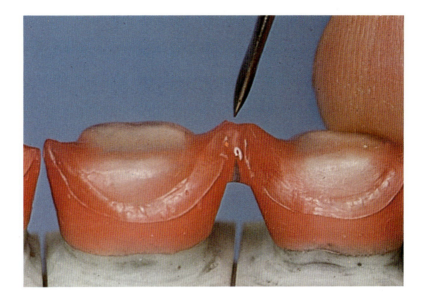

This illustration shows the formation of the wax connector between the molars.

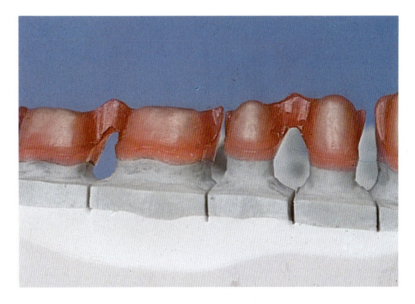

The finished wax connectors, buccal view.

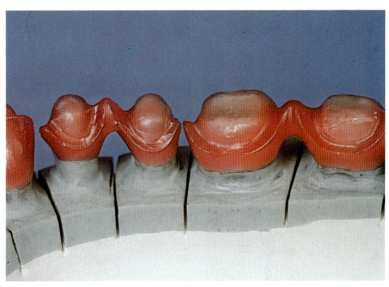

Lingual view of the connected molars and premolars.

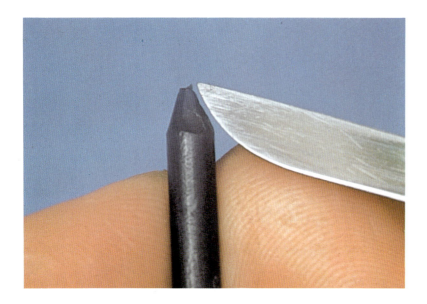

The wax sprue is fabricated. In this case, a wax rod with a 3.2mm diameter is used. The sprue is contoured coneshaped in order to compensate for casting pressure.

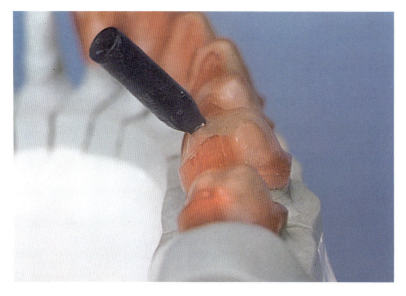

In consideration of the form, size, and thickness of a crown, the position of the sprue is located on the wax pattern in an area that guarantees the best casting results.

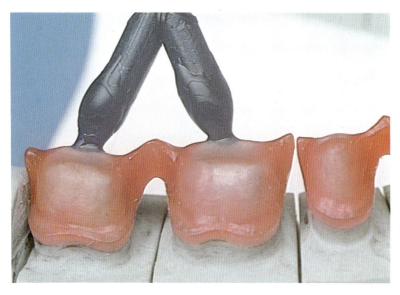

Here we choose the center of the occlusal surfaces.

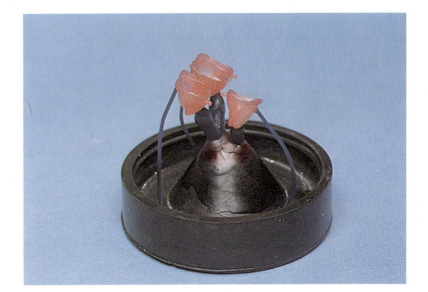

The wax patterns are luted to the sprueformer. Notice the angle and position of the wax patterns. Notice the placement of vents on the wax patterns and sprueformer.

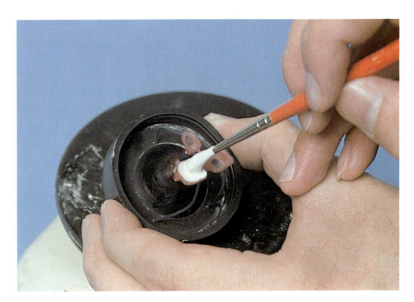

The investment material is mixed according to instructions from the manufacturer and applied with a camel hair brush to the wax patterns.

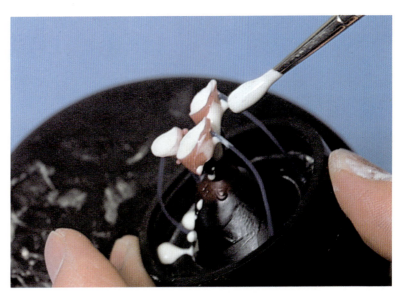

After applying some investment onto the exterior surfaces of the wax patterns, the investment is vibrated into the casting ring.

4.4 FINISHING AND ADJUSTING THE METAL CASTINGS

4.4.1. SELECTION OF THE CASTING ALLOY

In the preceding section, we discussed the wax-up procedure for the metal core portion of the ceramometal restoration.

In this section, we will demonstrate finishing and adjusting procedures for the metal casting, including contouring, provision of resistance form, and surface contour.

Only satisfactory completion of the procedures above will guarantee proper contour and coloring of the ceramometal restoration. The casting is finished in a standardized manner, using only a few selected stones.

If the metal core and/or the ceramometal restoration become distorted during the firing process or heat treatment, the restoration is worthless.

In the following section, seven foreign and Japanese ceramometal alloys frequently used for the construction of ceramometal restorations are discussed. Their changes during heat treatment are compared.

The metals from A to F contain Au as their main ingredient, being from 80 to 87% Au. The metal G contains 58.26% Au, 10.27% Pt, 29.54% Pd, and 1.93% Ru. at a high melting temperature of 1,460° C, thus indicated by the manufacturer.

The metals A to G represent test specimens which were cast with a centrifugal casting machine, using 0.5 x 5 x 20mm. sheet wax for the wax pattern. Although these products have more or less the same intrinsic properties, the degree of oxidation and other conditions differ greatly between them. This means that a chemical bond formed between porcelain and any one of these alloys is not necessarily uniform.

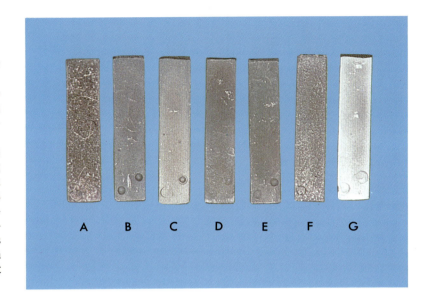

The photograph shows test specimens of A to F which have been heat treated at 1,000° C after completion of the casting process. Except for B and F, where no marked changes are visible to the naked eye, the other specimens show some alteration. The degree of oxidation is greatly influenced by changes due to heat treatment.

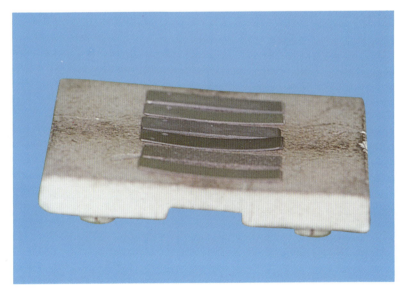

Test specimens A to F, after heat treatment at 1,000° C for 10 minutes, where only one side has been finished in a forward-backward motion in one direction only. Changes are noted on all the test specimens. Clearly, it is almost impossible to obtain a uniform oxidation film on the surface of any two of the tested specimens.

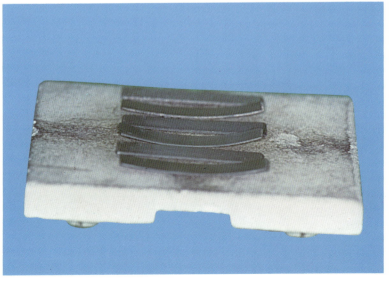

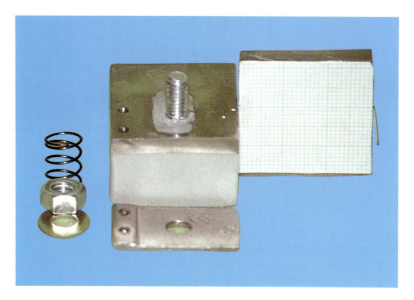

Testing equipment for the evaluation of heat changes in metal alloys.

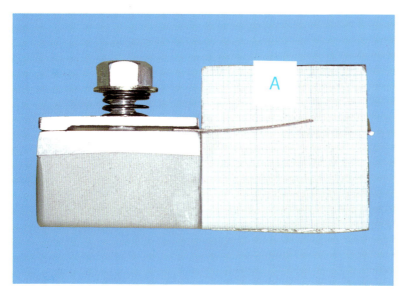

Test specimen A, heat treated at 1,000° C for 10 minutes. Only one side has been finished. After testing the degree of the heat change can be visually confirmed.

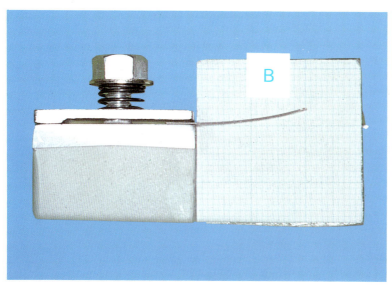

Test specimen B is similiarly tested.

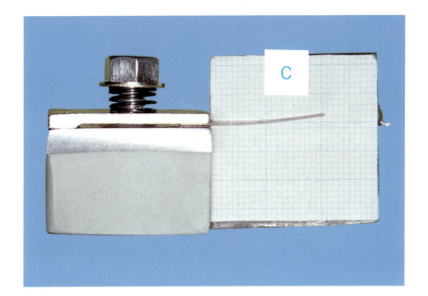

Test specimen C is similiarly tested.

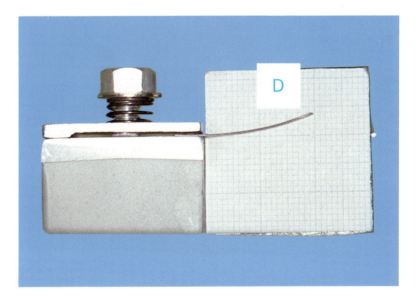

Test specimen D is similiarly tested.

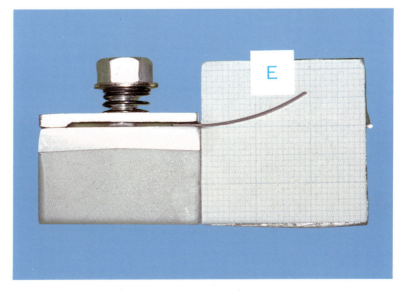

Test specimen E is similiarly tested.

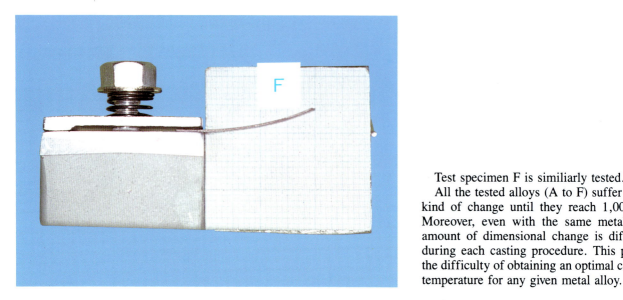

Test specimen F is similiarly tested.

All the tested alloys (A to F) suffer some kind of change until they reach 1,000° C. Moreover, even with the same metal, the amount of dimensional change is different during each casting procedure. This proves the difficulty of obtaining an optimal casting temperature for any given metal alloy.

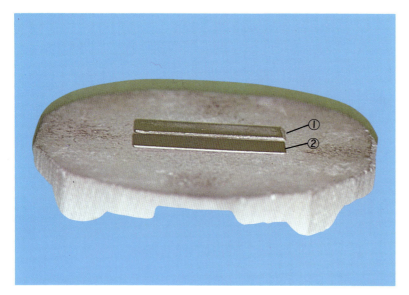

Test specimen G is heat treated at 1,066° C for 20 minutes. Side ① is unfinished and side ② is finished. There is no appreciable difference between the two.

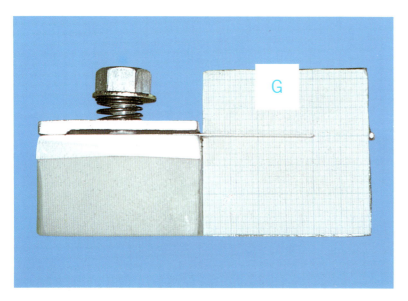

The second specimen is tested. When a metal alloy with a high melting temperature and the least possibility of oxidation is selected, a constantly stable condition can be obtained.

Metals A to F show a largely unstable chemical combination of porcelain and oxidation film. G, however, shows a stable mechanical combination of porcelain and bonding agent components.

When any one of the metals from A to F is selected, possible dimensional changes of the metal can be reduced through polishing the casting immediately after its heat treatment.

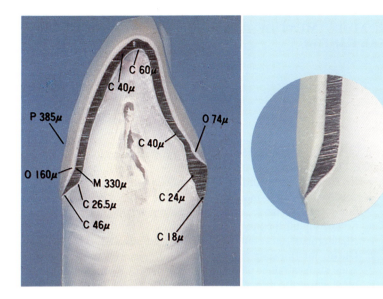

When metal G is used, there is no shrinkage of the porcelain as a result of baking, even when the tip of the margin is thin. The photograph shows a section of this test specimen with varying degrees of fit and thickness.

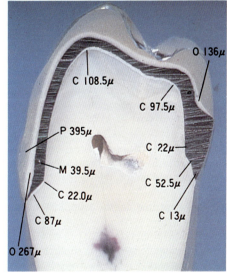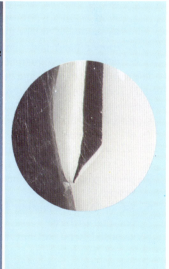

Here the margin area is thinner than in the illustration above, but there is no discernible metal distortion due to porcelain shrinkage after the firing process.

There are many possible reasons for the poor fit of any porcelain-metal crown. To avoid such problems, it is essential that a metal-alloy least susceptible to heat change be selected. In the process of adding the porcelain, we must avoid contaminating the inside of the casting with porcelain.

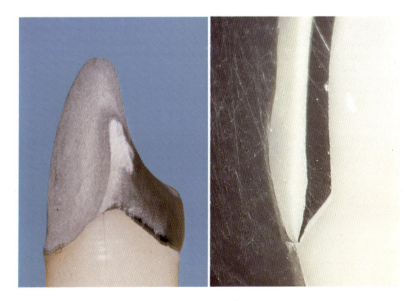

4.4.2. ADJUSTMENT OF THE METAL CASTING

A great variety of stones used for finishing and adjusting the casting are available. The author prefers a small standardized selection of stones and burs, which he chooses according to the following criteria:
1. A stone/bur which is most suitable for the task.
2. Within a feasible range, a larger size stone/bur is preferred.
   a. Proper digital manipulation
   b. Standardized procedure, established and adhered to
   c. During the finishing procedure, the handpiece should be moved in wide strokes rather than fast narrow strokes — this guarantees a more uniform surface appearance
   d. In order to minimize grinding, the contour must be well planned during the wax-up stage. If greater adjustments are needed, a large stone is initially used to create an even surface, and is then replaced by a smaller stone, more effective for minor adjustments.
   e. Proper hand and digital manipulation and exact control of rotational speed guarantee maximum proficiency.

The selection of stones and burs is based on the above criteria. The author usually uses Shofu Co. carborundum products for the grinding of cast restorations. The following burs are routinely used:
1. #48 carborundum point for narrow support areas.
2. #11 carborundum point for wide support areas.
3. #20 or 21 carborundum point for substructure surface.
4. #43 carborundum point for minor adustments of substructure surface.
5. #44 carborundum point for adjusting minor interdental papillary spaces.
6. #6 or 10 for adjusting areas between interdental pappillae and the occlusal surface.

For exposed metal portions, carborundum points (1) to (3) can be selected as indicated. For adjusting a narrow interdental area, a thin separator disk, also a Shofu Co. product, can be recommended.

For non-precious metal restorations such as Ni-Cr alloy, the same points can be used. But since this alloy is extremely hard to grind, we recommend the use of Faiot high strength points or Busch heatless stones.

For final polishing after adjustment of the substructure surface, the following can be used with precious and non-precious metals.

1. Fuji soft rubber wheel (Fuji Co.)
2. Silicon wheel (Shofu Co., available in three colors of black, brown and green)
3. GC silicon wheel (Brown)
4. GC silicon wheel (Gray)
5. Rubber wheel #61 (Dedeco Co. product)
6. Black and gray rubber wheels #17 (Dedeco Co. products)
7. P1-3 (Shofu Co. product)

Products (4) to (7) are recommended for non-precious metals. Product (3) is recommended for gross finishing procedures. Product (4) is recommended for the final finishing.

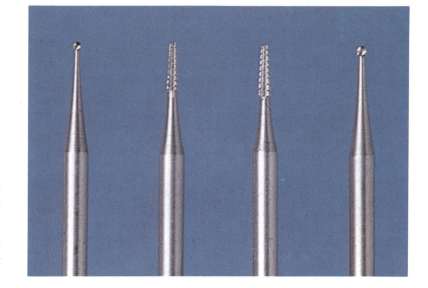

Although an internal adjustment of the metal structure is necessary, precision casting procedures minimize the necessity for subsequent adjustment. Spot adjustments inside a crown have to be kept to a minimum. The author usually uses the Jota or Busch burs for these minor adjustments.

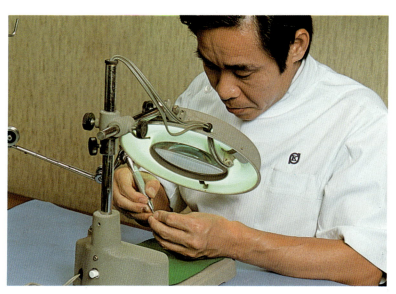

Minute discrepencies inside the crown are adjusted carefully under magnification.

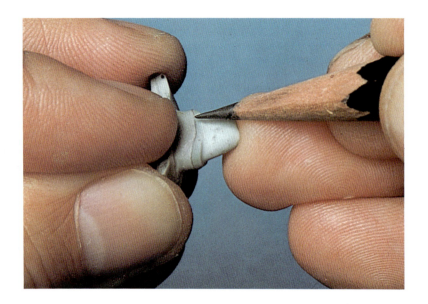

The marginal portions of the die are marked with a pencil prior to adjustment.

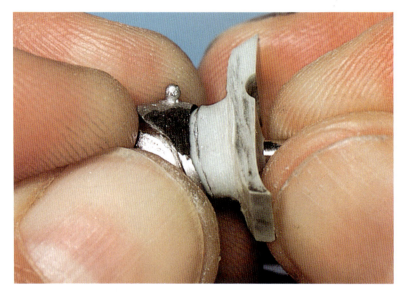

The crown is fitted onto the die to confirm exact fit.

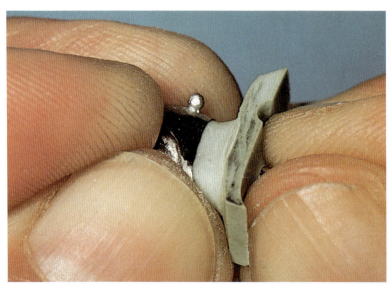

The above confirmation is made under magnification. Thus we can easily recognize marginal discrepencies.

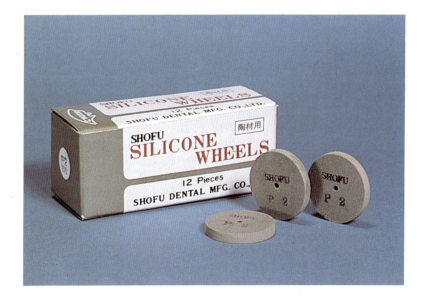

An adjustment of the marginal portion is made with a Shofu wheel (P-2.)

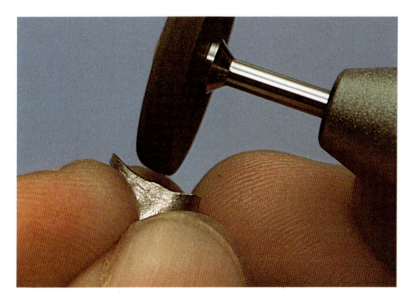

An adjustment of too-long margins is performed by holding the crown firmly in place so that it will not be damaged in the working process. Any adjustment is best accomplished under magnification.

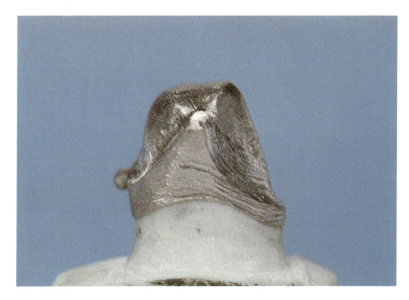

After the margins are adjusted, they are checked for proper lengths. Subsequently, adjustments of the support areas are made.

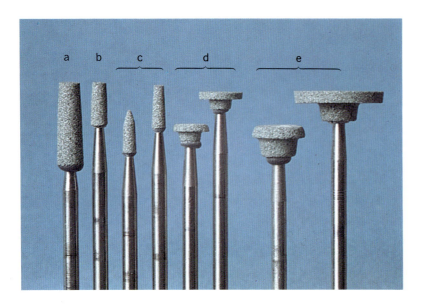

This set of 5 stones (Shofu carborundum products) are routinely used by the author. **a** : #20, **b** : #43, **c** : #44, **d** : #48, **e** : #11.

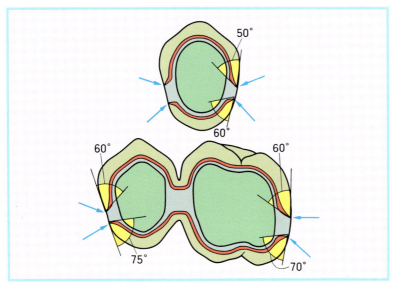

The angle of the support area is normally 70° (viewed horizontally) to prevent exposure of the opaque and to guarantee uniform procelain thickness. A suitable stone/bur is selected.

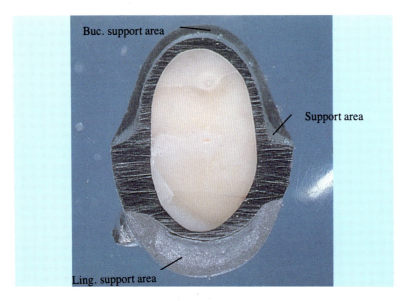

Buc. support area

Support area

Ling. support area

An occlusal view of the metal restoration after an adjustment to its support areas. Note the angle of the support area and its contour.

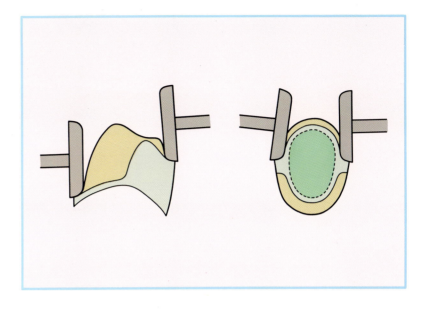

A correctly angled stone is most efficient during adjustment of the metal casting.

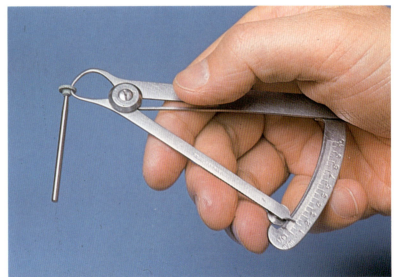

The angles of the stones #48 and #11 are adjusted to conform with the angle of the support area. The 0.9mm (#48) and 1.6mm (#11) stones provide us with working guides for the thickness of the porcelain to be added later.

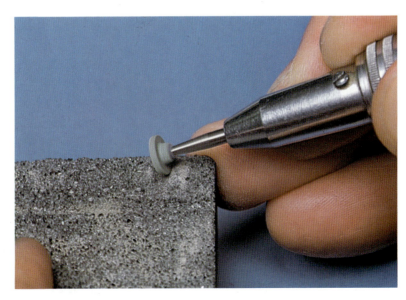

The #48 stone needs to be modified to conform with the angle of the support area. This modification must take into account the abrasion of the modified stone.

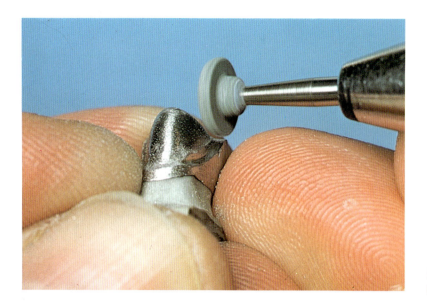

The buccocervical region of the metal casting of the first premolar, adjusted with a #48 stone.

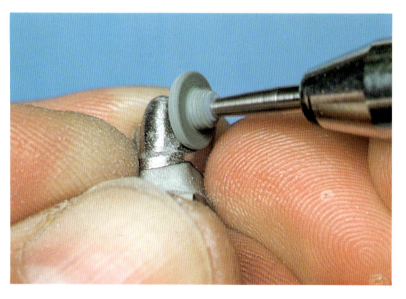

Here a large stone is used with a larger stroke at low speed, scribing a broad, smooth arc.

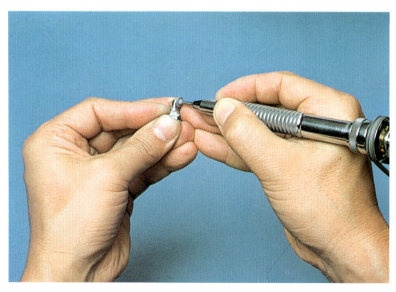

When a stone is used on the working model, the metal casting may be damaged by slight movements of the die. Therefore, a lock model is recommended for this process.

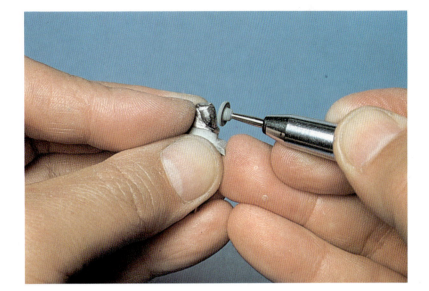

An adjustment is made at the buccal support area.

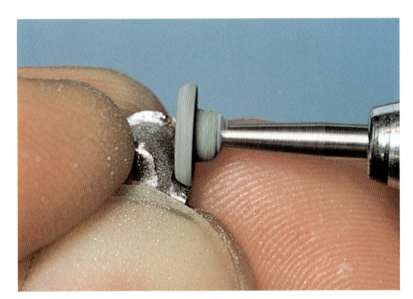

An adjustment is made in the proximal and buccal portion of the casting.

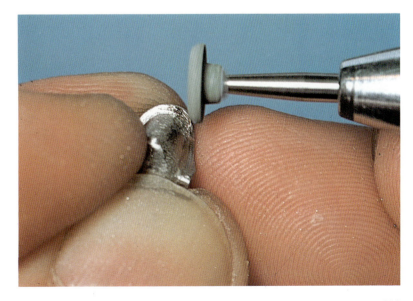

An adjustment effected in one continuous motion from the buccal to the distal proximal areas. We achieve this type of movement using one wide sweeping stroke, rather than small intermittent motions. The same principle applies for the lingual support area.

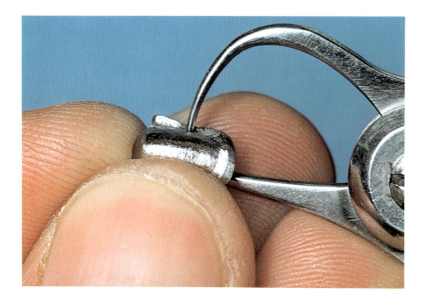

In the process of adjusting the support area, it is necessary to check for proper thickness of the casting using a gauge.

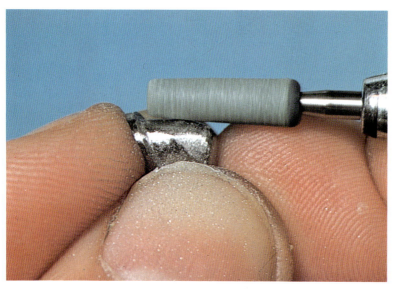

The #20 or #21 stone is used for grinding most of the metal surface except for the support areas in order for it to accept the ceramic material later, where an adjustment has already been completed. Here, the stone is brought into contact with the tip of the line angle of the support area and is gradually worked toward the occlusal surface of the casting.

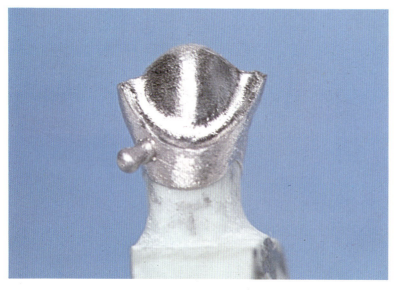

A lingual view of the maxillary first premolar on which all necessary adjustments have been completed.

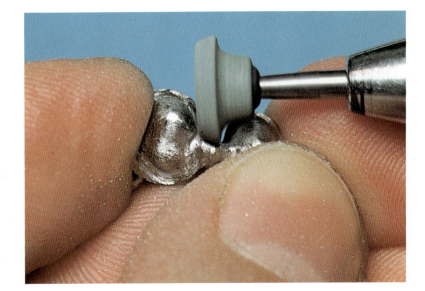

The solder joint is adjusted with a #48 stone. By using a large stone (#11), we can create a more uniform surface.

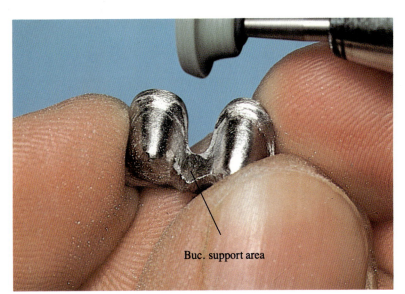

Buc. support area

A buccal view of the support area after the adjustment has been made. During the next step, we adjust the interdental portion of the solder joint.

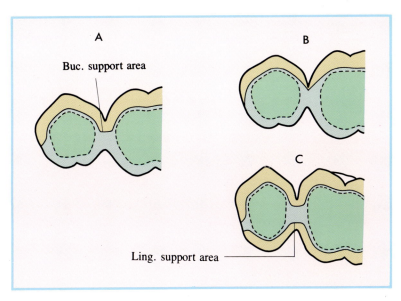

A

Buc. support area

B

C

Ling. support area

A and C in this illustration show well-adjusted solder joints, while B shows an incorrectly contoured rigid connector.

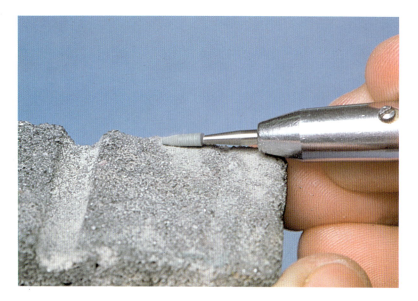

A #44 stone is used for the adjustment of an interdental papillary region on the rigid connector. Its tip needs to be modified to conform with the proximal form.

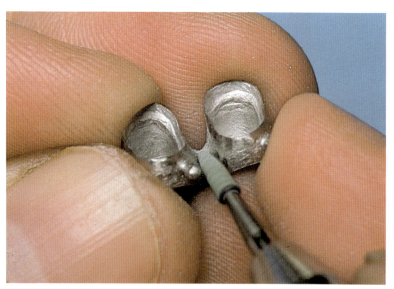

An adjustment is made in the area of the interdental papillary region, to the lingual surface of the solder joint.

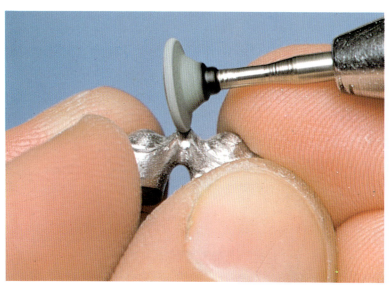

Subsequently, the lingual surface and rigid connector are adjusted, using either a #6 or #10 stone with a ball-like tip. A #10 stone has been used in this particular case. The adjustment is extended from the transition area to the interdental region.

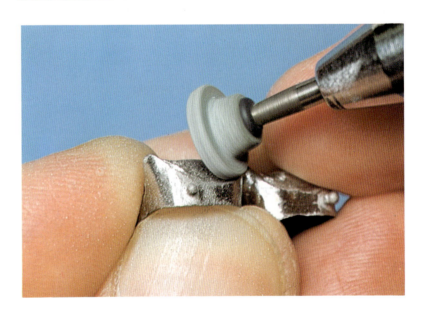

The support area on the lingual molar surface is adjusted with a #48 stone. With a large casting, a #11 stone, about 1.6mm thick, can also be used. The stone must be modified to match the U shape of this area.

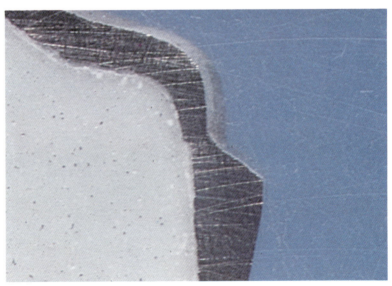

The lingual support area is adjusted. It is prepared sufficiently large to resist compressive forces exerted on the porcelain.

A section of the above after completed adjustments.

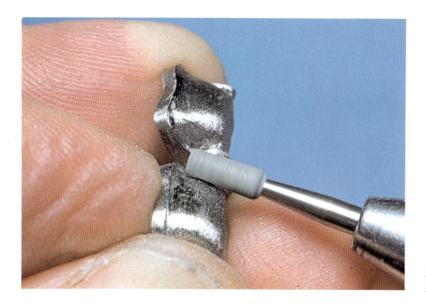

After all supporting areas have been adjusted, the metal substructure is finally adjusted with the #20 stone.

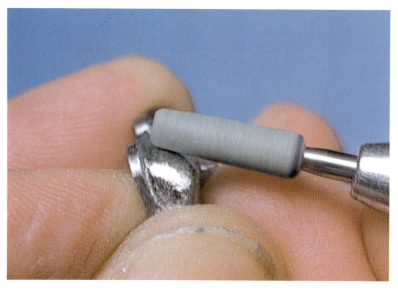

It is important in this process to prepare the entire surface as evenly as possible.

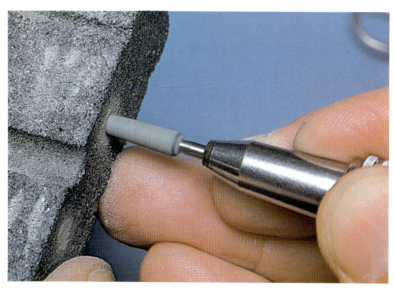

The exposed metal part is adjusted with either a #20 or #21 stone after modifying the stone's tip to a right angle.

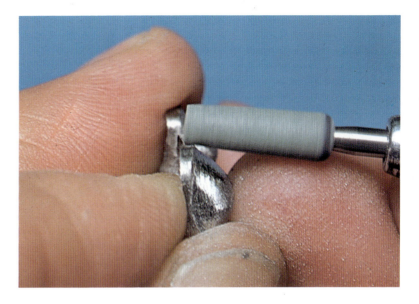

The exposed metal portion must be adjusted to form a smooth transition from the interdental area to the cervix. The stone should not touch the margin. Keep a distance of about 0.2mm. The remaining portion is polished after final completion of the porcelain.

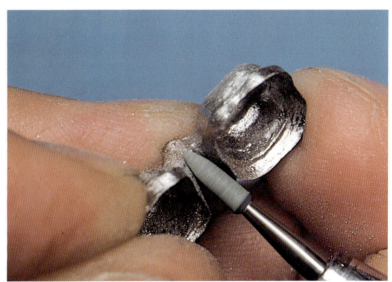

Here a #44 stone is used, and the same precautions are observed.

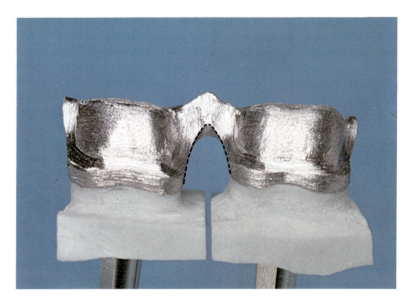

The buccal view of a metal casting with both mandibular molars connected. Note the well-contoured embrasure.

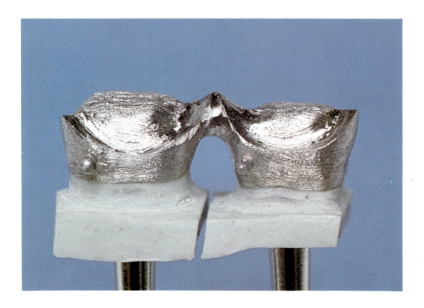

A lingual view of the same restoration. A U-shaped skeleton and trestle design can be observed in the solder joint area. Needless to say, the connectors of a fixed partial denture must be extremely strong.

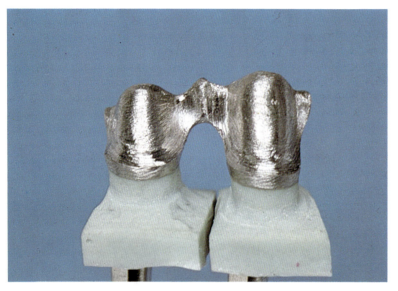

The buccal view of a restoration in which two castings are connected rigidly.

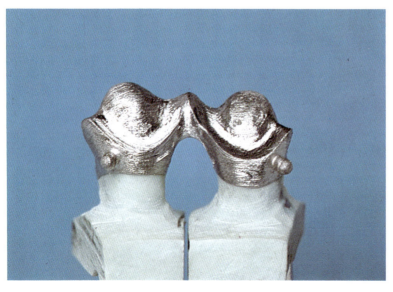

A lingual view of the same restoration. The lower boundary of the trestle is determined by the interdental papillae. In consideration of sufficient embrasure, ease of oral hygiene, and strength of the solder joint, the lingual support area of this restoration is prepared as needed. For this reason, the metal part on the top of the solderjoint is exposed.

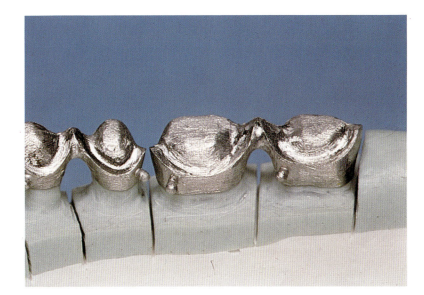

A lingual view of the restoration placed on its dies after necessary adjustments have been completed.

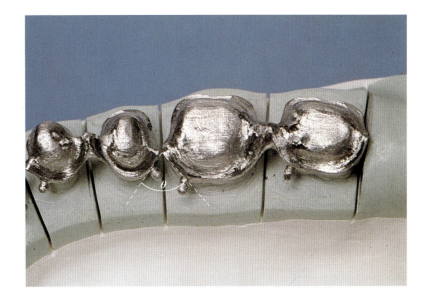

An occlusal view. Note that the forces exerted on the occlusal surfaces are absorbed by the peripheries of the support areas. The first and second premolars, now unconnected, are brought into contact with each other with porcelain later. The angle formed by the two lingual sides of the restoration plays an important role in the relationship of the two proximal surfaces.

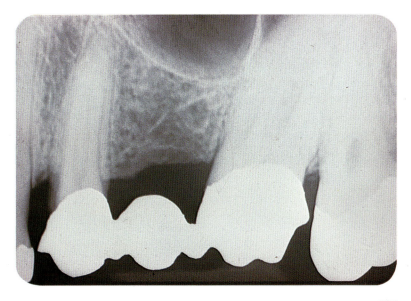

A radiograph of a restoration cemented in the mouth. The interdental papillae have been contoured as planned (photograph courtesy of Dr. R.S. Stein).

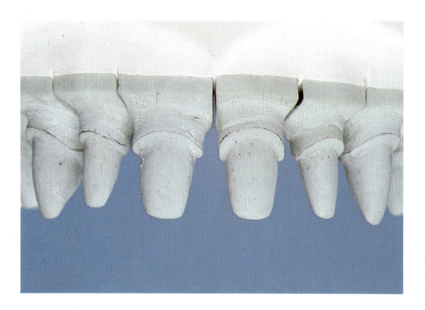

The labial view of the dies of the maxillary anterior teeth. The gingival margins here are prepared with a long chamfer of 70°.

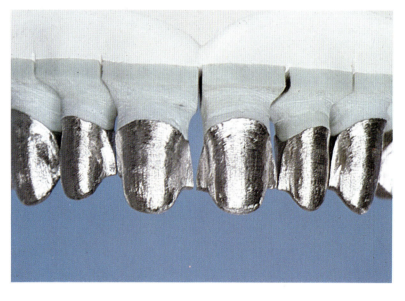

The maxillary anterior restorations are placed back on the dies. The lingual surfaces of these restorations will be covered with porcelain. Note the embrasure contours.

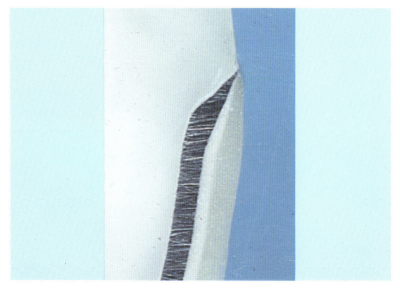

When preparing the gingival margin at an angle greater than 50°, the extreme end of the marginal portion can be covered with opaque and porcelain.

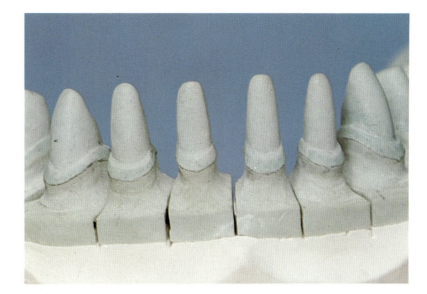

A labial view of the dies of the mandibular anterior teeth. The marginal areas are prepared as beveled chamfers.

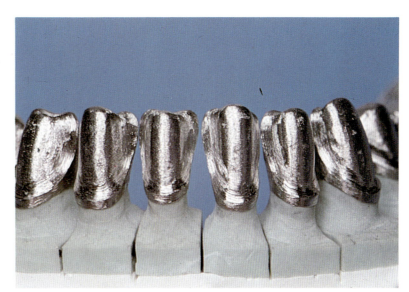

A labial view of the anterior castings placed on their dies. The proximal supporting areas are placed lingually.

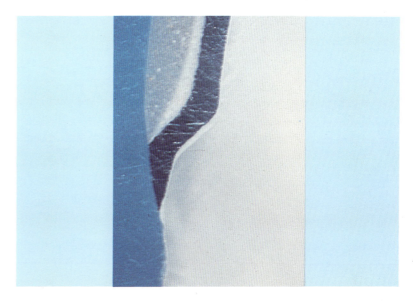

Since the gingival bevel of the mandibular anterior retainer is less than 50°, some metal exposure will occur in that area.

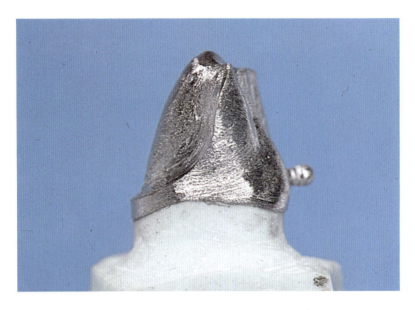

A mesial view of the mandibular canine casting, placed on its die. Note the proper width and angle of the support area. Note the curvature in the proximal contact area. A satisfactory proximal contour has been achieved.

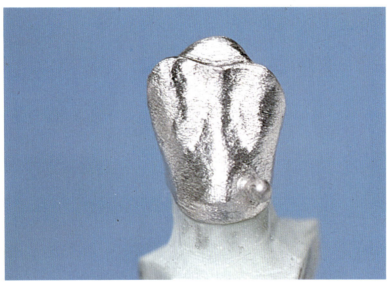

A lingual view of the same restoration.

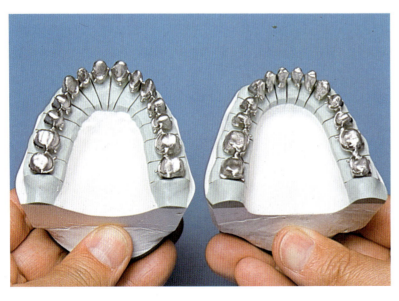

This view shows the maxillary and mandibular castings placed on their dies after the completed adjustment.

4.4.3 FINAL FITTING OF THE CASTINGS IN THE PATIENT'S MOUTH

During the construction of fixed partial dentures, especially ceramometal restorations, the castings are tried in the mouth prior to the firing and finishing of the porcelain.

The following points are checked:
a. Proper fit
b. The relation between gingival tissues and crown contour
c. Guarantee for sufficient porcelain thickness of the restorations, especially where they come in contact during mandibular movement
d. The triangular structure (metal, opaque, and porcelain) in relation to the gingival tissues
e. Confirmation of proper occlusal relationships

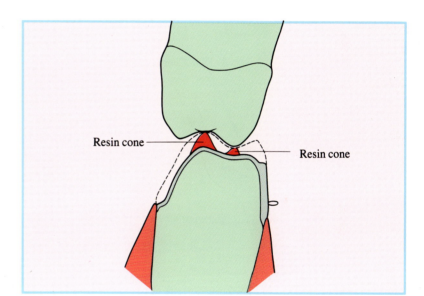

When opposing teeth are present, polymer resin cones are placed onto the occlusal surfaces of the mandibular castings. The tips of the cones are brought into contact with the marginal ridges or the lingual cusps of the maxillary teeth. These cones are the casting check cones.

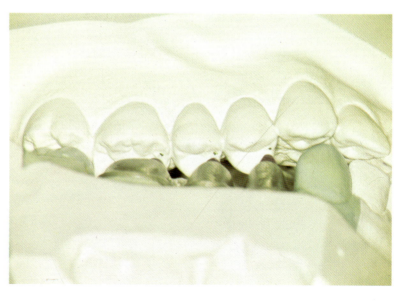

When placing the casting check cones, their contacts with the opposing teeth should be marked in pencil.

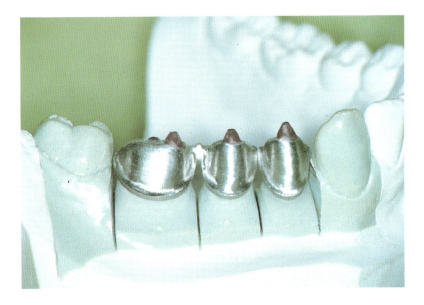

After the resin cones have set, their occlusal relations with the opposing teeth are checked, using a contact ribbon. The marked occlusal contacts are important. The cones are used as a working guide for confirmation of the accuracy of the mounted casts and dies.

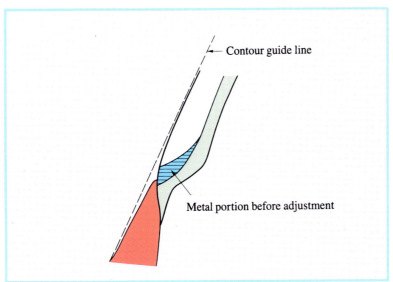

Contour guide line

Metal portion before adjustment

When the castings are tried in the mouth, a plaster impression is taken of the dies in situ. On the plaster impression, the relations between the gingival tissues and the castings are reproduced. If the cervical area of a casting cannot be clearly viewed, the height of the gingival tissues should be registered. Any information on the height of the gingival tissues helps in determining the amount of exposed metal in the cervical region.

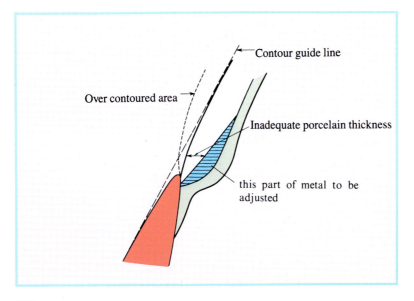

Contour guide line

Over contoured area

Inadequate porcelain thickness

this part of metal to be adjusted

The amount of porcelain which has to be built up in the cervical region of the crown can also give us information about the final contour of the restoration. When the occlusal surface is reproduced with porcelain, the dental laboratory needs a correct occlusal registration from the dentist. The dental technician is then able to restore the occlusal surface (of the restoration) precisely.

4.5 MANIPULATION OF THE BONDING AGENT

The bonding between metal and porcelain may be of any type or a combination of types among the following:

1. Mechanical bonding
2. Chemical bonding (chemical bonding between the metal surface and oxides contained in the porcelain)
3. Bonding through Van der Waals forces (mutal attraction of metal and porcelain electrons)
4. Compressive bonding (through the compressive strength of the porcelain)

Chemical bonding (2) is regarded as the most important type, and for this reason, various elements —including Sn, Fe, Ir, and In — are added to the metal, and the opaque contains Sn in the form of an oxide.

Heat treatment of the metal, prior to the porcelain build-up, functions as a degassing and oxidation treatment. The degree of oxidation plays an important role in this type of bonding. It is extremely difficult to produce the desired level of oxidation at a constant rate. In some cases, the porcelain may become separated from the metal alloy, due to lack of sufficient bonding. Since the maintenance of a constant level of oxidation is difficult to achieve even when using the same material, the difficulties are greater when different materials and equipment are employed.

If the fluctuation of those factors is permitted to influence laboratory procedures, a satisfactory restoration cannot be expected. Now a bonding agent has been developed which can largely compensate for the problems mentioned above. After the porcelain surface is coated with this bonding agent and then fired, platinum particles are retained on its surface. Thus we are able to obtain a stable type of mechanical bonding.

For this reason, the ideal metal (PI alloy) does not contain oxidized trace elements. It must be non-oxidizing. It must be processed at the high temperature of 1,460° C in order to prevent dimentional changes in the metal during the degassing process. For the same reason, we use PI porcelain which has a high coefficient of thermal expansion, compatible with that of the PI alloy and least susceptible to possible distortion.

When producing any type of mechanical bonding, porosities may be generated at the junction between the metal and porcelain. Yet when standard procedures are followed, there is no difference in the strength or esthetic appearance of the material. With the PI porcelain, the opaque particles are smaller than the platinum particles used in the bonding agent. Therefore, they are compatible and almost no porosities are found.

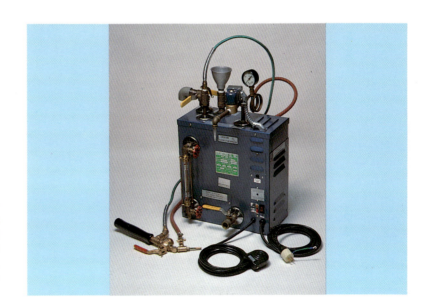

The occlusal relationship between the teeth of the maxillary and mandibular arches is examined. The previously constructed planning crowns and the functional guides assist us in this task.

After adjustments are completed, the castings are sand blasted. When working with precious metals, the use of a pointed tip is preferred since the restoration may otherwise be damaged during the sand blasting process. A high pressure steam cleaner is recommended to clean the restoration.

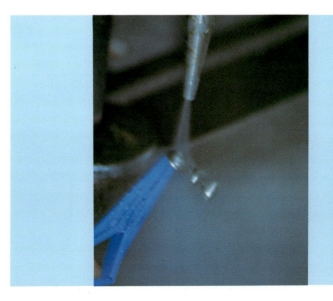

A good high pressure cleaner can be as effective as and is preferred to an acid cleaner. When cleaning the casting, it is placed approximately 3cm away from the steam outlet. The dies are simultaneously cleaned.

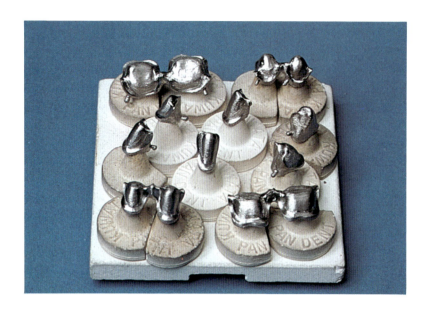

Restorations which have been cleaned with the high pressure steam apparatus. After the cleaning, the restoration should not be contaminated through finger contact.

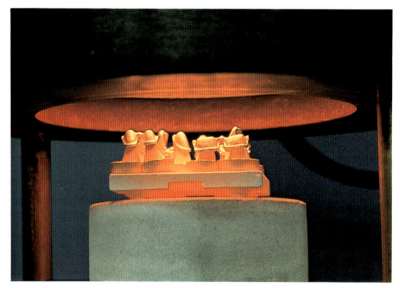

In order to eliminate voids and to burn impurities, the restoration should be heat treated. Since the P1 metal used in this case is non-oxidizing, there is no need to effect the oxide treatment. The PI metal is heat treated, exposing it to air at a temperature of 1,066° C, for 15 to 20 minutes.

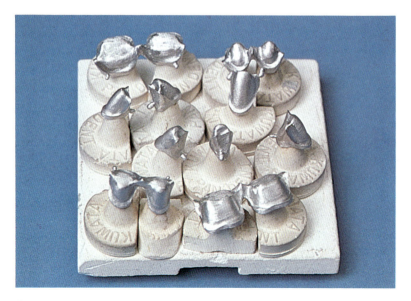

The photograph shows the result of the heat treatment. Since the fusing temperature of the PI metal is 1,460° C, the restoration does not suffer from dimensional heat changes. Since this metal is non-oxidizing, the application of the bonding agent and the baking are carried out prior to the subsequent process of porcelain build-up.

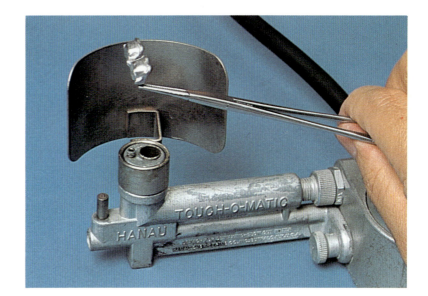

Before applying the bonding agent to the casting, the metal is heated over the flame of a Bunsen burner.

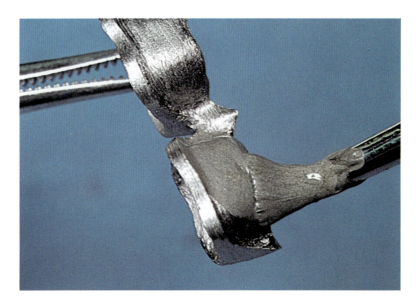

The bonding agent (KPD) is available in paste form. It contains gold, platinum, and a pine resin with fatty oils. Because of the oils the paste fails to adhere to metal if it does not reach a high enough temperature. It is necessary to heat the bonding agent adequately in order to obtain sufficient adhesion (Particle size of the platinum is 3 micron.).

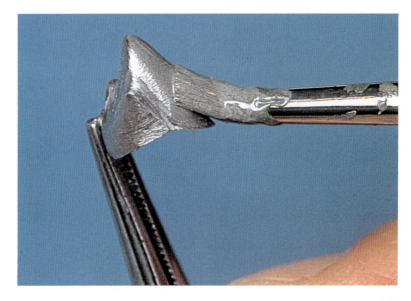

For application of the bonding agent, a hard brush is recommended. The bonding agent is applied only on the metal surfaces which will receive porcelain. When applied too thickly, the agent may accumulate in drops in the cervical region and become ineffective. Holding the casting at its marginal area should be avoided.

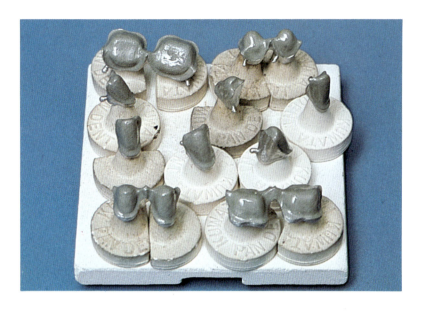

Here we see a group of castings with the bonding agent applied.

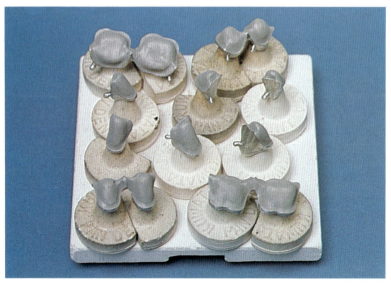

The heating of the bonding agent takes 15 minutes at a temperature of 1,066° C. This temperature must be maintained throughout the process in order to guarantee proper adhesion of porcelain to the metal casting. If the temperature is lower, the platinum particles will not adhere to the surface firmly enough to produce the desired bond strength. At this temperature, the pine resin and other paste ingredients are completely burnt out.

In its upper portion, this view shows a metal surface of a casting with the bonding agent applied evenly; the lower view shows a surface finished with a stone only. Note the even distribution of the platinum particles in the upper fired surface.

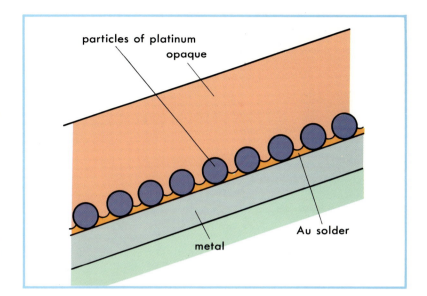

A schematic illustration of a sectioned ceramometal restoration with the bonding agent applied. The platinum particles are only approximately 3 micron in diameter.

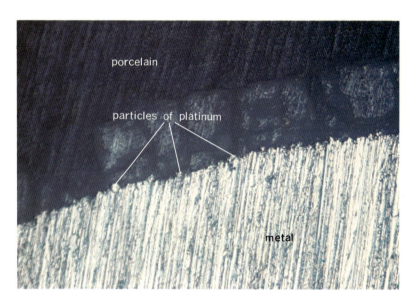

A micrograph of a sectioned surface with the bonding agent applied. Note the absence of porosities on the surface.

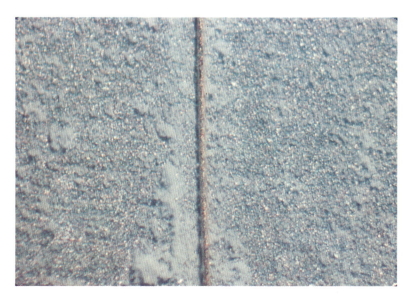

Another micrograph of a sectioned surface with the bonding agent applied. In the center we see a wire of a 25 micron diameter. The sparkling spots in this view are the platinum particles (diameter: 3 microns). Fine porcelain particles are located in the interstices of the platinum particles; thus the bonding surface and the strength of the restoration increase. Clearly, the porcelain particles must be combined properly in order to guarantee sufficient bond strength and strength of the final restoration.

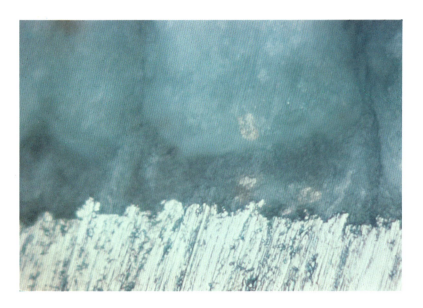

Another micrograph of a sectioned metal surface with the bonding agent applied and fired. Note the close relationship of the platinum and porcelain particles. The platinum particles which act as retentive elements increase the final strength of the restoration.

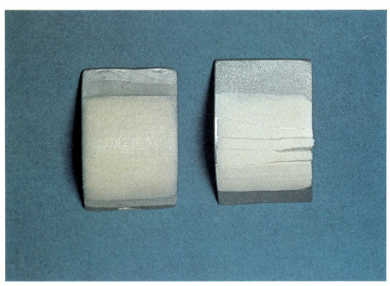

Since the PI alloy is of a non-oxidizing nature, chemical bonding from an oxidation film between the metal and porcelain is not expected, but it is essential to use some type of bonding agent for the PI alloy in order to obtain the needed strength. If this is neglected, the porcelain may exfoliate as shown on the right side.

A view of a 0.3mm thick PI metal plate which is folded. Since it has been strengthened by usng a bonding agent, crazing can be detected, yet the porcelain does not exfoliate.

Thus the use of a bonding agent guarantees sufficient strength for the final ceramometal restoration.